Psychiatric Disorders and Diabetes Mellitus

Psychiatric Disorders and Diabetes Mellitus

Edited by

Maria D Llorente MD
Julie E Malphurs PhD

Mental Health and Behavioral Science Service
Miami VA Healthcare System
Department of Psychiatry and Behavioral Science
Miller School of Medicine at the University of Miami
Miami, FL
USA

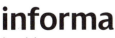

informa

healthcare

First published in the United Kingdom in 2007 by Informa Healthcare, 4 Park Square, Milton Park, Abingdon, Oxon OX14 4RN. Informa Healthcare is a trading division of Informa UK Ltd. Registered office, 37/41 Mortimer Street, London W1T 3JH. Registered in England and Wales number 1072954.

Tel: +44 (0)20 7017 6000
Fax: +44 (0)20 7017 6336
Email: info.medicine@tandf.co.uk
Website: www. informahealthcare.com

A CIP record for this book is available from the British Library.
Library of Congress Cataloging-in-Publication Data

Data available on application

ISBN-10: 0 415 38541 5
ISBN-13: 978 0 415 38541 1

Distributed in North and South America by
Taylor & Francis
6000 Broken Sound Parkway, NW, (Suite 300)
Boca Raton, FL 33487, USA

Within Continental USA
Tel: 1 (800) 272 7737; Fax: 1 (800) 374 3401
Outside Continental USA
Tel: (561) 994 0555; Fax: (561) 361 6018
Email: orders@crcpress.com

Distributed in the rest of the world by
Thomson Publishing Services
Cheriton House
North Way
Andover, Hampshire SP10 5BE, UK
Tel: +44 (0)1264 332424
Email: tps.tandfsalesorder@thomson.com

Composition by C&M Digitals (P) Ltd, Chennai, India
Printed and bound in India by Replika Press Pvt Ltd

Contents

List of contributors   vii

1. Overview of diabetes mellitus   1
   Jennifer B Marks

2. Diabetes mellitus and schizophrenia   17
   Oscar Villaverde

3. Diabetes mellitus and depression   29
   Julie E Malphurs

4. Diabetes mellitus and cognitive impairment   41
   José A Luchsinger and Hermes Florez

5. Diabetes mellitus and sexual dysfunction   53
   Marilyn Sanjuan-Horvath

6. Diabetic peripheral neuropathic pain: an inevitable
   consequence of diabetes mellitus?   75
   B Eliot Cole and Maria D Llorente

7. HIV-1 infection, diabetes mellitus, and psychiatric
   disorders   89
   Karl Goodkin, Stephen Symes, Mauricio Concha,
   Michael Kolber, Deshratn Asthana, Rebeca Molina, Alicia
   Frasca, Wenli Zheng, Sandra O'Mellan, and Maria del Carmen
   Lichtenberger

8. Nutritional interventions for individuals with mental
   illness and diabetes mellitus   115
   Louise Z Grant

9.   Impact of exercise on psychiatric disorders and
     diabetes mellitus   131
     Neva J Kirk-Sanchez

10. Psychopharmacologic treatment of psychiatric
     disorders in patients with diabetes mellitus: clinical
     considerations and options   153
     Jose A Rey

11. Treatment options for diabetic peripheral
     neuropathic pain   179
     Maria D Llorente and B Eliot Cole

12. Psychosocial therapies for psychiatric
     disorders and diabetes mellitus   195
     *Alan M Delamater, Jessica M Valenzuela,
     and Michelle M Castro*

13. Collaborative care to improve treatment of
     co-occurring diabetes mellitus and
     psychiatric disorders   219
     Maria D Llorente and Jesica Soto

Index   239

Contributors

Deshratn Asthana PhD
Department of Psychiatry and
   Behavioral Sciences
Miller School of Medicine at
   the University of Miami
Miami, FL
USA

Michelle M Castro BS
Department of Pediatrics
Mailman Center for Child
   Development
Miller School of Medicine
   at the University
   of Miami
Miami, FL
USA

B Eliot Cole MD MPA
American Society of Pain
   Educators
Montclair, NJ
USA

Mauricio Concha MD
Department of Neurology
Miller School of Medicine at
   the University of Miami
Miami, FL
USA

Alan M Delamater PhD
Department of Pediatrics
Miller School of Medicine at
   the University of Miami
Miami, FL
USA

**Maria del Carmen
   Lichtenberger** PSYD
Department of Psychiatry and
   Behavioral Sciences
Miller School of Medicine at
   the University of Miami
Miami, FL
USA

Hermes Florez MD MPH
Geriatric Research, Education
   and Clinical Center
Miller School of Medicine at
   the University of Miami
Veterans Affairs Medical Center
Miami, FL
USA

Alicia Frasca PSYD
Department of Psychiatry and
   Behavioral Science
Miller School of Medicine at
   the University of Miami
Miami, FL
USA

Karl Goodkin MD PhD
Department of Psychiatry
   and Behavioral Sciences,
   Neurology and Psychology
Miller School of Medicine at
   the University of Miami
Miami, FL
USA

Louise Zang Grant PhD RD
Nutrition and Food Service
Miami VA Healthcare System
Miami, FL
USA

Neva J Kirk-Sanchez PT PhD
Department of Physical
   Therapy
Miller School of Medicine at
   the University of Miami
Coral Gables, FL
USA

Michael Kolber PhD, MD
Clinical Immunology
   Department of Internal
   Medicine Infectious Diseases
   Division
Jackson Memorial Hospital
Miller School of Medicine at
   the University of Miami
Miami, FL
USA

Maria D Llorente MD
Mental Health and Behavioral
   Science Service
Miami VA Healthcare System
Department of Psychiatry and
   Behavioral Science
Miller School of Medicine at
   the University of Miami
Miami, FL
USA

José A Luchsinger MD MPH
Division of General
   Medicine
Department of Medicine
Taub Institute for Research on
   Alzheimer's Disease and the
   Aging Brain
Columbia University
New York, NY
USA

Julie E Malphurs PhD
Mental Health and Behavioral
   Science Service
Miami VA Healthcare
   System
Department of Psychiatry and
   Behavioral Science
Miller School of Medicine
   at the University
   of Miami
Miami, FL
USA

Jennifer B Marks MD
Division of Endocrinology,
   Diabetes and Metabolism
Miller School of Medicine at
   the University of Miami
Diabetes Management
   Program
Miami VA Medical Center
Miami, FL
USA

Rebeca Molina MD MPH
Department of Psychiatry and
    Behavioral Sciences
Miller School of Medicine at
    the University of Miami
Miami, FL
USA

Sandra O'Mellan AS
Department of Psychiatry and
    Behavioral Sciences
Miller School of Medicine at
    the University of Miami
Miami, FL
USA

Jose A Rey PharmD
Pharmaceutical and
    Administrative Sciences
Nova Southeastern University
College of Pharmacy
Ft. Lauderdale, FL
USA

Marilyn Sanjuan-Horvath MD
Mental Health and Behavioral
    Science Service
Miami VA Healthcare System:
    Department of Psychiatry and
    Behavioral Science
Jackson Memorial Hospital
Miller School of Medicine at
    the University of Miami
Miami, FL
USA

Jesica Soto RD
Miami VA Healthcare System
Miami, FL
USA

Stephen Symes MD
Department of Internal
    Medicine
Division of Infectious Diseases
Miller School of Medicine at
    the University of Miami
Miami, FL
USA

Jessica M Valenzuela MS
Department of Pediatrics
Mailman Center for Child
    Development
Miller School of Medicine at
    the University of Miami
Miami, FL
USA

Oscar Villaverde MD
Mental Health and Behavioral
    Science Service
Miami VA Healthcare System;
    Department of Psychiatry and
    Behavioral Science
Miller School of Medicine at
    the University of Miami
Miami, FL
USA

Wenli Zheng MS
Department of Psychiatry and
    Behavioral Sciences
Miller School of Medicine at
    the University of Miami
Miami, FL
USA

Chapter 1

Overview of diabetes mellitus

Jennifer B Marks

Diabetes mellitus

Definition

Diabetes mellitus (DM) is actually a group of metabolic disorders characterized by hyperglycemia which can result from defects in insulin secretion, insulin action, or both. Chronic hyperglycemia is associated with the development of damage to various organs in the body – the eyes, kidneys, nervous system, and cardiovascular system.

Epidemiology

DM and its complications constitute a significant public health problem worldwide, and are an important cause of morbidity and mortality. In fact, DM has reached epidemic proportions throughout the world, and the prevalence numbers are expected to continue to rise. Worldwide there were 194 million adults with DM in 2003, and this number is expected to reach 333 million by the year 2025, with many cases developing in poorer, developing countries.[1] A rise in obesity rates over the past decade is to blame for much of the increase in type 2 DM. Today, nearly two-thirds of US adults are overweight or obese.[2] It has been projected that one in three US citizens born in 2000 will develop DM.[3]

The risk of developing DM rises not only with obesity (body mass index [BMI] $\geq 25\,\text{kg/m}^2$) and lack of physical activity but also with increasing age (≥ 45 years) and family history. Specific population subgroups have a higher prevalence of DM than the population as a whole.[4] For example, type 2 DM is more common in African-Americans, Hispanic Americans, Native Americans, Asian Americans, and Pacific Islanders. Women with a history of prior gestational DM or polycystic ovarian syndrome are at increased risk. Risk factors for the development of DM include hypertension, dyslipidemia (high-density lipoprotein [HDL] cholesterol ≤35 mg/dl and/or triglyceride level ≥250 mg/dl), vascular disease, impaired glucose tolerance (IGT), or impaired fasting glucose (IFG). The greater the number of risk factors present in an individual, the greater the chance of that individual developing diabetes.

Classification and pathogenesis

Type 1 DM, previously known as insulin-dependent DM, is most often the result of an autoimmune, destructive process targeting the β-cells of the pancreas, usually leading to absolute insulin deficiency.[4] It becomes clinically apparent when 80–90% of the insulin-secreting cells are destroyed. The great proportion of people with DM (90–95%), however, have type 2 DM.[5]

There are two underlying mechanisms which lead to the onset of clinical type 2 DM: inadequate insulin action in target tissues (insulin resistance) and inadequate secretion from pancreatic β-cells[6] (Figure 1.1). Insulin resistance arises prior to the onset of clinical disease, but predicts the development of DM.[7–9] Environmental factors, particularly obesity and a sedentary lifestyle, are important contributors to the development of DM, largely because of their effects on insulin sensitivity.[10–12] When target tissues become insulin resistant, glucose uptake is decreased, hepatic glucose production increases, and lipolysis is enhanced. In muscle, the increased free fatty acid (FFA) availability accelerates fat oxidation, resulting in decreased insulin-mediated glucose uptake and disposal. In the liver, elevated FFAs promote gluconeogenesis and increase hepatic glucose output.

When inadequate insulin secretion from β-cell dysfunction is also present, hyperglycemia develops, heralding the onset of type 2 DM.[6–9] In the natural history of progression to DM, β-cells initially increase insulin secretion in response to insulin resistance, and for a period of time are able to effectively maintain glucose levels below the DM range. However, when β-cell function begins to decline, insulin production is inadequate to overcome the insulin resistance, and blood glucose levels rise. Insulin resistance, once established, remains relatively stable over time. Therefore, progression of DM is a result of worsening β-cell function with pre-existing insulin resistance.

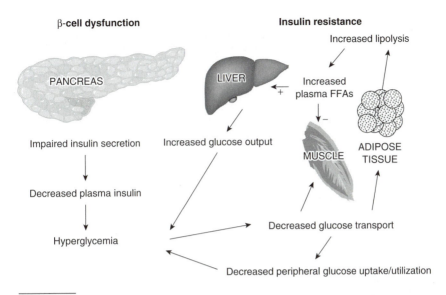

Figure 1.1   *Defects in the pancreas and in target tissues for insulin action in type 2 DM. In the non-diabetic individual, insulin suppresses hepatic glucose output, stimulates glucose uptake and utilization in muscle and adipose tissue, and suppresses lipolysis in adipose tissue. When these tissues become resistant to the actions of insulin, hepatic glucose production increases, glucose uptake is decreased, and lipolysis is enhanced. Increased free fatty acids (FFAs) from lipolysis stimulate cellular uptake of FFAs and lipid oxidation. In muscle, the increased FFA availability accelerates fat oxidation, resulting in decreased insulin-mediated glucose uptake and utilization. In the liver, elevated FFAs stimulate gluconeogenesis and increase hepatic glucose output. When β-cell dysfunction is present, insulin resistance in the target tissues leads to hyperglycemia and the development of type 2 DM. (Adapted from DeFronzo,[6] with permission.)*

Diagnosis

The diagnostic criteria for DM and the two high-risk categories of pre-DM, i.e. IFG and IGT, are defined in Table 1.1.[4] There are three ways to diagnose DM. Because of simplicity of use, acceptability to patients, and low cost, the fasting plasma glucose (FPG) is the preferred diagnostic test. In the presence of symptoms of DM (polyuria, polydipsia, weight loss, etc.), a casual plasma glucose of >200 mg/dl is diagnostic. The 75 g oral glucose tolerance test (OGTT) is more sensitive and modestly more specific than FPG, but it is poorly reproducible and rarely performed in clinical settings.

In the absence of unequivocal hyperglycemia, any test used to diagnose DM must be confirmed on a subsequent day by a plasma glucose

Table 1.1   The diagnostic criteria for diabetes and the classification of impaired fasting glucose (IFG) and impaired glucose tolerance (IGT)

	FPG (mg/dl)	2-H PG (mg/dl)	Sx of Diabetes + CPG
Normal	<100	<140	–
IFG	≥100 and <126	–	–
IGT	–	≥140 and >200	–
Diabetes	≥126	≥200	+ and CPG ≥200 mg/dl

FPG, fasting plasma glucose. 2-HPG, 2-hour post 75 g glucose load plasma glucose. CPG, casual plasma glucose. Sx (symptoms) of diabetes: polydipsia, polyuria, and weight loss.

Adapted from American Diabetes Association Position Statement,[4] with permission.

measured either in the fasting state or 2 hours after an oral glucose load. The use of the hemoglobin A_{1c} (HbA_{1c}) for the diagnosis of DM is not recommended, as it is less specific and assays are not completely standardized throughout the world.

Hyperglycemia insufficient to meet the diagnostic criteria for diabetes is categorized as either IFG or IGT, depending on whether it is identified by an FPG or an OGTT. Impaired fasting glucose is diagnosed when the FPG level is ≥100 mg/dl but <126 mg/dl. IGT exists when the plasma glucose level 2 hours after a 75 g oral glucose load is ≥140 mg/dl but <200 mg/dl. These are considered to be pre-DM states.

Screening

Screening to detect pre-DM (IFG or IGT) and DM should be considered in individuals ≥45 years of age, particularly in those with a BMI ≥25 kg/m². Screening should also be considered for people who are <45 years of age and are overweight if they have another risk factor for DM. Repeat testing should be carried out at 3-year intervals.[4]

Goals of treatment: prevention of complications

Chronic poor glycemic control is associated with the development of DM vascular complications, including microvascular (retinopathy, neuropathy, and nephropathy) and macrovascular (premature cardiovascular disease [CVD]). CVD (coronary and cerebrovascular) is the cause of 65% of deaths in patients with type 2 DM.[13] Epidemiologic studies have shown that the risk of a myocardial infarction (MI) or CVD death in a DM individual with no prior history of CVD is comparable to that of an individual who has had a previous MI.[14,15]

Microvascular complications can be delayed or prevented by maintaining excellent chronic glycemic control, as has been demonstrated in a number of interventional trials, including the Diabetes Control and Complications Trial (DCCT), the United Kingdom Prospective Diabetes Study (UKPDS), the Kumamoto Study, and the Stockholm Diabetes Intervention Study.[16–22] Further, even in acute illness, several studies have shown that intensive insulin therapy and improved glycemic control are associated with better outcomes.[23,24]

Intensive glycemic control also results in reduced macrovascular complications, i.e. CVD, as demonstrated in a number of epidemiologic studies.[25–27] Direct randomized clinical trial evidence of the impact of improved glycemic control on macrovascular complications is accumulating. From the Diabetes Control and Complications Trail/Epidemiology of Diabetes Interventions and Complications (DCCT/EDIC) Study of type 1 DM, it is clear that intensive glycemic control prior to the onset of vascular disease has long-term beneficial effects on the risk of CVD in this population.[28] In the UKPDS, a 16% reduction in the risk of MI, including non-fatal and fatal MI and sudden death, was observed in the cohort of type 2 DM subjects randomized to tight blood glucose control, a trend towards statistical significance.[20] A secondary multivariate observational analysis of the 10-year follow-up data of this original UKPDS cohort showed that for every 1% reduction in hemoglobin A_{1c} (HbA_{1c}), there was a 14% decrease in fatal and non-fatal MI.[29] Similar risk reduction was shown in a secondary multivariate observational analysis of systolic blood pressure.[30] Based on results from clinical trials of glycemic control and the impact on DM microvascular complications, recommendations for targets of glycemic control have been put forward.[4,31]

Diabetes management

Glycemic goals

Glycemic control is fundamental to the management of diabetes. The HbA_{1c} is the most accepted indicator of chronic control, reflecting

Table 1.2 Glycemic goals	
HbA$_{1c}$ goal *for patients in general*	<7%
HbA$_{1c}$ goal *for the individual patient*	<6% (as close to normal as possible)
Preprandial capillary plasma glucose[a]	90–130 mg/dl
Peak postprandial capillary plasma glucose[a]	<180 mg/dl

[a]Capillary plasma glucose = fingerstick glucose.

Adapted from American Diabetes Association Position Statement,[4] with permission.

fasting and postprandial glucose concentrations. The goal of therapy is to achieve an HbA$_{1c}$ as close to normal as possible in the absence of hypoglycemia. Recommended glycemic goals for non-pregnant individuals are shown in Table 1.2. Less stringent treatment goals may be appropriate for patients with limited life expectancies, in the very young or older adults, and in individuals with comorbid conditions. Severe or frequent hypoglycemia is an indication for the modification of treatment regimens, including setting higher glycemic goals.

More stringent goals (i.e. a normal HbA$_{1c}$ <6%) should be considered in individual patients based on epidemiologic analyses suggesting that there is no lower limit of HbA$_{1c}$ at which further lowering does not reduce the risk of complications, but further HbA$_{1c}$ lowering is associated with risk of increased hypoglycemia (particularly in those with type 1 DM). However, the absolute risks and benefits of lower targets are unknown. The risks and benefits of stringent vs less stringent control in type 2 DM are currently being tested in two ongoing studies: the Action to Control Cardiovascular Risk in Diabetes (ACCORD) trial[32] and the VA Cooperative Study on Glycemic Control and Complications in Diabetes Mellitus – Type 2.[33]

Strategies for achieving glycemic goals

Nutrition and physical activity

Overweight and obesity are strongly linked to the development of type 2 DM and can complicate its management. Moderate weight loss improves glycemic control and reduces CVD risk. Therefore, weight loss is an important therapeutic strategy in all overweight or obese individuals who have type 2 DM. All patients with type 2 DM should be encouraged to maintain a healthy lifestyle by exercising and following an appropriate diet.[34] The primary approach for achieving

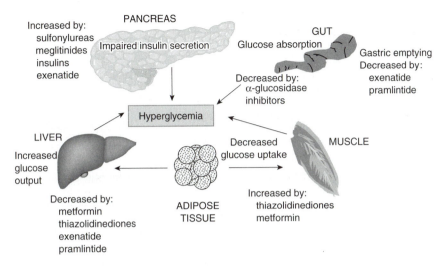

Increased by:
sulfonylureas
meglitinides
insulins
exenatide

PANCREAS

Impaired insulin secretion

GUT

Glucose absorption

Gastric emptying
Decreased by:
exenatide
pramlintide

Decreased by:
α-glucosidase
inhibitors

Hyperglycemia

LIVER

Increased
glucose
output

Decreased
glucose uptake

MUSCLE

Decreased by:
metformin
thiazolidinediones
exenatide
pramlintide

ADIPOSE
TISSUE

Increased by:
thiazolidinediones
metformin

Pramlintide also increases satiety via CNS mechanisms

Figure 1.2 *Antidiabetic agents and their mechanisms of action. The variety of antidiabetic agents for the treatment of type 2 DM target different mechanisms in the underlying pathogenesis of the disease. Sulfonylureas and the meglitinides (repaglinide, nateglinide) are insulin secretagogues that stimulate release of insulin from the pancreas. Metformin, a biguanide, improves insulin sensitivity chiefly by reducing insulin resistance in the liver, thereby decreasing hepatic glucose production. The thiazolidinediones (rosiglitazone, pioglitazone) improve insulin sensitivity primarily in the muscle, thereby increasing peripheral uptake and utilization of glucose. The α-glucosidase inhibitors (acarbose, miglitol) prevent the breakdown of carbohydrates to glucose in the gut, by inhibiting the enzymes that catalyze this process, thereby delaying carbohydrate absorption. Insulin and insulin analogues increase insulin levels in the presence of declining β-cell function and diminished endogenous insulin secretion. Exenatide and the synthetic amylin pramlintide exploit novel mechanisms related to effects on glucagon secretion, gastric emptying, and satiety. (Adapted from DeFronzo[35] and White JR and Campbell K,[36] with permission.)*

weight loss is therapeutic lifestyle change, which includes a reduction in energy intake and an increase in physical activity. In type 1 DM, a balanced diet is important for maintaining equilibrium between insulin requirements and energy intake and expenditure.

Oral antidiabetic agents

A variety of antidiabetic pharmaceutical agents for the treatment of type 2 diabetes are available; they target different mechanisms in the underlying pathogenesis of the disease[4,35,36] (Figure 1.2). There are five

Table 1.3 Available oral antidiabetic agents

Drug class	Mechanism of action	Major side effects
Sulfonylureas Meglitinides	Stimulate insulin secretion	Weight gain Hypoglycemia
Metformin	Suppress hepatic glucose production (major) Improve insulin sensitivity in target tissues (minor)	GI side effects Lactic acidosis (rare)
Thiazolidinediones	Improve insulin sensitivity in target tissues (major) Suppress hepatic glucose production (minor)	Weight gain Edema Congestive heart failure
α-Glucosidase inhibitors	Delay carbohydrate absorption from the intestine	Flatulence or abdominal discomfort

categories of oral agents on the market, which can be used initially in most cases of type 2 DM, until insulin deficiency becomes severe and insulin replacement is required. Sulfonylureas and the meglitinides (repaglinide, nateglinide) are insulin secretagogues that stimulate release of insulin from the β-cells of the pancreas. Metformin, a biguanide, improves insulin sensitivity chiefly by reducing insulin resistance in the liver, thereby decreasing hepatic glucose production. The thiazolidinediones (rosiglitazone, pioglitazone) improve insulin sensitivity primarily in the muscle, thereby increasing peripheral uptake and utilization of glucose. The α-glucosidase inhibitors (acarbose, miglitol) prevent the breakdown of carbohydrates to glucose in the gut, by inhibiting the enzymes that catalyze this process, thereby delaying carbohydrate absorption. One of the sulfonylureas or metformin are a usual first choice for pharmacologic treatment, and have equal efficacy to lower HbA_{1c} by approximately 1–1.5% as monotherapy. However, most patients will eventually require treatment with combinations of oral medications with different mechanisms of action simultaneously in order to attain adequate glycemic control. Table 1.3 lists the available classes of oral antidiabetic medications, their mechanisms of action, and side effects.

Injectable therapy

Injectable agents for treatment of type 1 or type 2 DM include traditional insulin preparations, newer insulin analogues, amylin, and incretin mimetics (see Figure 1.2). Insulin and the insulin analogues increase circulating insulin levels in the presence of declining β-cell function and diminished endogenous insulin secretion. Insulin and analogues, available in both long-acting and rapid-acting formulations, can be used in combination with oral agents in type 2 DM, or as insulin replacement therapy in type 1 and longstanding, insulin-deficient type 2 DM. The recent additions to the market – the incretin mimetic exenatide and the synthetic amylin pramlintide – exploit novel mechanisms related to effects on glucagon secretion, gastric emptying, and satiety to improve glycemic control.

Strategies for achieving non-glycemic goals

In addition to hyperglycemia, individuals with type 2 DM often have a constellation of other metabolic abnormalities that increase their CVD risk.[30,37–41] Risk determinants of CVD include the presence or absence of coronary heart disease (CHD), other clinical forms of atherosclerotic disease, and the major risk factors: high low-density lipoprotein (LDL) cholesterol, cigarette smoking, hypertension (>130/>80 mmHg), low HDL cholesterol, family history of premature CHD (defined as a relative with CHD <65 years old for women and <55 years old for men), and age (men ≥45 years old, women ≥55 years old). Note that diabetes is considered to be a CHD equivalent, so the goal for LDL cholesterol is <100 mg/dl. Based on these risk determinants, the Expert Panel on Detection, Evaluation, and Treatment of High Blood Cholesterol in Adults (Adult Treatment Panel III) identifies three categories of risk that modify the goals and modalities of LDL-lowering therapy (Tables 1.4 and 1.5).[42]

Risk reduction strategies have been demonstrated to be highly effective in a number of studies. The Multiple Risk Factor Intervention Trial (MRFIT), performed in 347 978 men aged 35–57 years old, demonstrated that the absolute risk of CVD death was approximately three times higher for men with DM than for those without DM, regardless of age, ethnic background, and risk factor level.[43] In the UKPDS, CHD risk factors were evaluated by inclusion in a Cox proportional hazards model.[44] In order of impact, and all statistically significant, were LDL cholesterol, HDL cholesterol, HbA_{1c}, and systolic blood pressure.

The MICRO-HOPE Study included 3577 individuals with type 1 and 2 DM, with and without hypertension, and compared the cardiovascular event rates with the angiotensin-converting enzyme (ACE) inhibitor

Table 1.4   ATP III classification of LDL, total and HDL cholesterol (mg/dl)[a]

LDL cholesterol:	
<100	Optimal
100–129	Near optimal
130–159	Borderline high
160–189	High
≥190	Very high
Total cholesterol:	
<200	Optimal
200–239	Borderline high
≥240	High
HDL cholesterol:	
<40	Low
≥60	High

[a]ATP, Adult Treatment Panel; LDL, low-density lipoprotein; HDL, high-density lipoprotein.

Adapted from Expert Panel on Detection, Evaluation, and Treatment of High Blood Cholesterol in Adults (Adult Treatment Panel III),[42] with permission.

Table 1.5   Three categories of risk that modify LDL cholesterol goals

Risk category	LDL goal (mg/dl)
CHD and CHD risk equivalents	<100
Multiple (2+) risk factors	<130
0–1 risk factor	<160

CHD, coronary heart disease. DM is a CHD equivalent.

Adapted from Expert Panel on Detection, Evaluation, and Treatment of High Blood Cholesterol in Adults (Adult Treatment Panel III),[42] with permission.

ramipril vs placebo.[45] The results showed that treatment with ramipril lowered the risk of the primary outcome of combined MI, stroke, or CVD mortality by 25%, MI by 22%, stroke by 33%, and cardiovascular death by 37%. Lowering serum cholesterol has been demonstrated in many studies to be effective at reducing CVD risks, both as primary and secondary prevention. Recent studies have questioned whether even more aggressive LDL cholesterol lowering in high-risk individuals should be the appropriate target of such treatment.[46,47]

An important recent study used a focused, multifactorial intervention with strict targets and individualized risk assessment in patients with type 2 DM and microalbuminuria who were at increased risk for

Table 1.6   Summary of recommendations for adults with diabetes

Glycemic control:	
HbA$_{1c}$	< 7.0%^{a}
Preprandial capillary plasma glucose	90–130 mg/dl (5.0–7.2 mmol/L)
Peak postprandial capillary plasma glucose	<180 mg/dl (<10.0 mmol/L)
Blood pressure	<130/80 mmHg
Lipids:	
LDL	<100 mg/dl (<2.6 mmol/L)
Triglycerides	<150 mg/dl (<1.7 mmol/L)
HDL	>40 mg/dl (>1.1 mmol/L)

^{a}The HbA$_{1c}$ goal *for the individual patient may be* <6% (as close to normal as possible).
Adapted from American Diabetes Association Position Statement,[4] with permission.

macrovascular and microvascular complications. These data suggest that a long-term, targeted, intensive intervention involving multiple risk factors reduces the risk of both cardiovascular and microvascular events by about 50% among these patients. The advantages of a multifactorial approach to the reduction of cardiovascular risk are obvious. The challenge remains to ensure that this approach can be widely adopted[48] (Table 1.6).

Prevention or delay of type 2 diabetes mellitus

Another study which used a focused, multifaceted strategy utilized in individuals at high risk for type 2 diabetes has demonstrated that the onset of clinical disease can be delayed or prevented.[49] The Diabetes Prevention Program (DPP) was a 27-center randomized controlled trial that included 3234 people with IGT, randomized to placebo, metformin (850 mg twice daily), or a lifestyle-modification program with the goals of at least a 7% weight loss and at least 150 minutes of physical activity per week followed for an average of 2.8 years. After approximately 3 years of follow-up, the results demonstrated a 58% reduction in the incidence of DM development in the intensive lifestyle group vs a 31% reduction in the incidence of DM development in the metformin group, both highly statistically significant compared with the placebo group. About 45% of the participants were from minority groups (e.g. African-American, Hispanic), and 20% were ≥60 years old.

Type 2 DM prevention trials using other forms of pharmacological therapy have also reported a significant lowering of the incidence of diabetes. The α-glucosidase inhibitor acarbose reduced the risk by 32% in the STOP-NIDDM trial,[50] and the thiazolidinedione troglitazone reduced the risk by 56% in the TRIPOD study.[51] There are also data to suggest that blockade of the renin–angiotensin system[52] may lower the risk of developing DM, but more studies are necessary before these drugs can be recommended for preventing DM.

Psychosocial screening

Basic assessment of psychosocial status should be included as part of the medical management of DM. Psychosocial screening should include patient attitudes about illness, expectations for medical care and outcomes, affect/mood, general and diabetes-related quality of life, available resources (financial, social, and emotional), and psychiatric history. It is best to incorporate psychological assessment into routine care rather than wait for identification of a specific problem or a deterioration in psychological status. Opportunities for screening of psychosocial status occur at diagnosis, during regularly scheduled management visits, during hospitalizations, at discovery of complications, or at the discretion of the clinician when problems in glucose control, or adherence are suspected or identified.

Need for improving diabetes care

Standards of care for diabetes recommended by the American Diabetes Association are revised periodically and published yearly in the journal *Diabetes Care*. The implementation of the standards of care has been suboptimal in most clinical settings. A report[53] from the National Health and Nutrition Examination Survey (NHANES) 1999–2000 and NHANES III surveys demonstrated that only 37% of US adults with diabetes achieved an HbA_{1c} of <7%, only 36% had a blood pressure <130/80 mmHg, and only 48% had a cholesterol <200 mg/dl. Only 7.3% had overall 'good control', i.e. attained target goals for all vascular risk factors. Another study addressing quality of diabetes care in the USA[54] showed that during 1988–1995 there was a gap between recommended diabetes care (HbA_{1c} <7%, annual dilated eye examination, annual foot examination, evaluation for urine albumin or protein excretion and achieving blood pressure and lipid goals) and the care that patients actually received. In that study, only 28.8% of diabetics even had an HbA_{1c} measurement, 63.3% reported a dilated eye examination, and 54.8% had had a foot examination within the previous year; 18% of these diabetic individuals had an $HbA_{1c} > 9.5\%$.

Although many interventions to improve adherence to the recommended standards have been implemented, providing uniformly effective DM care remains a challenge. Education of health professionals and patients alike is one key to better success. Improved access to health care and education for all is critical. Multidisciplinary teams are ideal to provide care for people with chronic conditions such as DM and to encourage patients to become involved in appropriate disease self-management. Cooperative efforts between health care providers, health policy experts, public health officials and patients are needed to change the climate and outcomes for individuals with DM and at risk for DM in the USA.

References

1. American Diabetes Association, North American Association for the Study of Obesity, American Society for Clinical Nutrition. Weight management using lifestyle modification in the prevention and management of type 2 diabetes: rationale and strategies. Diabetes Care 2004; 27: 2067–73.
2. Ogden CL, Flegal KM, Carroll MD et al. Prevalence and trend in overweight among U.S. children and adolescents, 1999–2000. JAMA 2002; 288: 1728–32.
3. Mokdad AH, Serdula MK, Dietz WH et al. The spread of the obesity epidemic in the U.S. JAMA 1999; 282: 1519–22.
4. American Diabetes Association Position Statement. Standards of medical care for diabetes. Diabetes Care 2006; 29(Suppl 1): S4–42.
5. Harris MI, Flegal KM, Cowie CC et al. Prevalence of diabetes, impaired fasting glucose, and impaired glucose tolerance in U.S. adults. The Third National Health and Nutrition Examination Survey, 1988–1994. Diabetes Care 1998; 21: 518–24.
6. DeFronzo RA. Lilly lecture 1987. The triumvirate: beta-cell, muscle, liver. A collusion responsible for NIDDM. Diabetes 1988; 37: 667–87.
7. Weyer C, Tataranni PA, Bogardus C et al. Insulin resistance and insulin secretory dysfunction are independent predictors of worsening of glucose tolerance during each stage of type 2 diabetes development. Diabetes Care 2000; 24: 89–94.
8. Kahn S. The importance of β-cell failure in the development and progression of type 2 diabetes. J Clin Endocrinol Metab 2001; 86: 4047–58.
9. Weyer C, Bogardus C, Mott D et al. The natural history of insulin secretory dysfunction and insulin resistance in the pathogenesis of type 2 diabetes mellitus. J Clin Invest 1999; 104: 787–94.
10. Mokdad AH, Ford ES, Bowman BA et al. Diabetes trends in the U.S. 1990–1998. Diabetes Care 2000; 23: 1278–83.

11. Choi B, Shi F. Risk factors for diabetes mellitus by age and sex: results of the national population health survey. Diabetologia 2001; 44: 1221–31.
12. Hu F, Manson J, Stamfer M et al. Diet, lifestyle, and the risk of type 2 diabetes in women. N Engl J Med 2001; 345: 790–7.
13. Geiss LS, Herman WH, Smith PJ. Mortality in non-insulin dependent diabetes. In: Diabetes in America, 2nd edn. National Diabetes Data Group, NIH, NIDDK, 1995; NIH Pub No. 95-1468: 233–57.
14. Malmberg K, Yusuf S, Gerstein HC et al. Impact of diabetes on long-term prognosis in patients with unstable angina and non-Q-wave myocardial infarction: results of the OASIS (Organization to Assess Strategies for Ischemic Syndromes) Registry. Circulation 2000; 102: 1014–19.
15. Haffner SM, Lehto S, Rönnemaa T et al. Mortality from coronary heart disease in subjects with type 2 diabetes and in nondiabetic subjects with and without prior myocardial infarction. N Engl J Med 1998; 339: 229–34.
16. The Diabetes Control and Complications Trial Research Group. The effect of intensive treatment of diabetes on the development and progression of long-term complications in insulin-dependent diabetes mellitus. N Engl J Med 1993; 329: 977–86.
17. The Diabetes Control and Complications Trial/Epidemiology of Diabetes Interventions and Complications Research Group. Retinopathy and nephropathy in patients with type 1 diabetes four years after a trial of intensive therapy. N Engl J Med 2000; 342: 381–9.
18. The Diabetes Control and Complications Trial Research Group. Effect of intensive therapy on the development and progression of diabetic nephropathy in the Diabetes Control and Complications Trial. Kidney Int 1995; 47: 1703–20.
19. Steffes MW, Molitch M, Chavers BM et al for the Diabetes Control and Complications Trial/Epidemiology of Diabetes Interventions and Complications Study Group. Sustained reduction in albuminuria six years after the Diabetes Control and Complications Trial. Diabetes 2001; 50: A63.
20. United Kingdom Prospective Diabetes Study Group. Effect of intensive blood glucose control with sulfonylurea or insulin compared with conventional treatment and risk of complications in patients with type 2 diabetes. Lancet 1998; 352: 837–53.
21. Ohkubo Y, Kishikawa H, Araki E et al. Intensive insulin therapy prevents the progression of diabetic microvascular complications in Japanese patients with non-insulin-dependent diabetes mellitus: a randomized prospective 6-year study. Diabetes Res Clin Pract 1995; 28: 103–17.
22. Reichard P, Pihl M, Rosenqvist U et al. Complications in IDDM are caused by elevated blood glucose level: the Stockholm Diabetes Intervention Study (SDIS) at 10-year follow up. Diabetologia 1996; 39: 1483–8.
23. Malmberg K, Ryden L, Efendic S et al. Randomized trial of insulin–glucose infusion followed by subcutaneous insulin treatment in diabetic patients with acute myocardial infarction (DIGAMI study): effects on mortality at 1 year. J Am Coll Cardiol 1995; 26: 57–65.
24. Van den Berghe G, Wouters P, Weekers F et al. Intensive insulin therapy in critically ill patients. N Engl J Med 2001; 345: 1359–67.
25. Coutinho M, Gerstein HC, Wang Y et al. The relationship between glucose and incident cardiovascular events: a meta-regression analysis of published data from 20 studies of 95 783 individuals followed for 12.4 years. Diabetes Care 1999; 22: 233–40.
26. Khaw KT, Wareham N, Luben R et al. Glycated hemoglobin, diabetes, and mortality in men in Norfolk cohort of European Prospective Investigation of Cancer and nutrition (EPIC-Norfolk). BMJ 2001; 322: 15–18.

27. Ostrander LD Jr, Lamphiear DE, Block WD, Williams GW, Carman WJ. Physiological variables and diabetic status. Findings in Tecumseh, Mich. Arch Intern Med 1980; 140: 1215–19.

28. The Diabetes Control and Complications Trial/Epidemiology of Diabetes Interventions and Complications Study Research Group. Intensive diabetes treatment and cardiovascular disease in patients with type 1 diabetes. N Engl J Med 2005; 353: 2643–53.

29. Stratton IM, Adler AI, Neil HAW et al for the UK Prospective Diabetes Study Group. Association of glycemia with macrovascular and microvascular complications of type 2 diabetes (UKPDS 35): prospective observational study. BMJ 2000; 321: 405–12.

30. Adler AI, Stratton IM, Neil HA et al for the UK Prospective Diabetes Study Group. Association of systolic blood pressure with macrovascular and microvascular complications of type 2 diabetes (UKPDS 36): prospective observational study. BMJ 2000; 321: 412–19.

31. AACE Medical Guidelines for the management of diabetes mellitus. American Diabetes Association Position Statement. Standards of medical care for patients with diabetes mellitus. Diabetes Care 2002; 25: 213–29.

32. Action to Control Cardiovascular Risk in Diabetes (ACCORD) Trial. http://www. clinicaltrials.gov/ct/show/NCT00000620?order=1.

33. Abraira C, Duckworth W, McCarren M et al for the participants of the VA cooperative study on glycemic control and complications in diabetes mellitus type 2. Design of the cooperative study on glycemic control and complications in diabetes mellitus type 2: Veterans Affairs Diabetes Trial. J Diabetes Complications 2003; 17: 314–22.

34. Nathan DM. Initial management of glycemia in type 2 diabetes mellitus. N Engl J Med 2002; 347: 1342–9.

35. DeFronzo RA. Pharmacologic therapy for type 2 diabetes. Ann Intern Med 1999; 131: 281–303.

36. White JR, Campbell K. Recent developments in the pharmacological reduction of blood glucose in patients with type 2 diabetes. Clin Diabetes 2001; 19: 153–9.

37. Ginsberg HN. Insulin resistance and cardiovascular disease. J Clin Invest 2000; 106: 453–8.

38. Hsueh WA, Law RE. Cardiovascular risk continuum: implications of insulin resistance and diabetes. Am J Med 1998; 105: 4S–14S.

39. Meigs JB, Mittleman MSA, Nathan DM et al. Hyperinsulinemia, hyperglycemia and impaired homeostasis. The Framingham Offspring Study. JAMA 2000; 283: 221–8.

40. Cooper ME, Bonnet F, Oldfield M et al. Mechanisms of diabetic vasculopathy: an overview. Am J Hypertens 2001; 14: 475–86.

41. Brownlee M. Biochemistry and molecular cell biology of diabetic complications. Nature 2001; 414: 813–20.

42. Expert Panel on Detection, Evaluation, and Treatment of High Blood Cholesterol in Adults (Adult Treatment Panel III). Executive summary of the third report of the National Cholesterol Education Program Expert Panel on detection, evaluation, and treatment of high blood cholesterol in adults. JAMA 2001; 285: 2486–97.

43. Stamler J, Vaccaro O, Neaton JD et al. Diabetes, other risk factors, and 12-yr cardiovascular mortality for men screened in the Multiple Risk Factor Intervention Trial. Diabetes Care 1993; 16: 434–44.

44. Turner RC, Millns H, Neil HA et al. Risk factors for coronary artery disease in non-insulin dependent diabetes mellitus: United Kingdom Prospective Diabetes Study (UKPDS: 23). BMJ 1998; 316: 823–8.

45. Heart Outcomes Prevention Evaluation Study Investigators. Effects of ramipril on cardiovascular and microvascular outcomes in people with diabetes mellitus: results of the HOPE study and MICRO-HOPE substudy. Lancet 2000; 355: 253–9.

46. Collins R, Armitage J, Parish S et al for the Heart Protection Study Collaborative Group. MRC/BHF Heart Protection Study of cholesterol-lowering with simvastatin in 5963 people with diabetes: a randomised placebo-controlled trial. Lancet 2003; 361: 2005–16.

47. Cannon CP, Braunwald E, McCabe CH et al. Intensive versus moderate lipid lowering with statins after acute coronary syndromes. N Engl J Med 2004; 350: 1495–504.

48. Gaede P, Vedel P, Larsen N et al. Multifactorial intervention and cardiovascular disease in patients with type 2 diabetes. N Engl J Med 2003; 348: 383–93.

49. The Diabetes Prevention Program Research Group. Reduction in the incidence of type 2 diabetes with lifestyle intervention or metformin. N Engl J Med 2002; 346: 393–403.

50. Chiasson JL, Josse RG, Gomis R et al. Acarbose for prevention of type 2 diabetes mellitus: the STOP-NIDDM randomised trial. Lancet 2002; 359: 2072–7.

51. Buchanan TA, Xiang AH, Peters RK et al. Preservation of pancreatic β-cell function and prevention of type 2 diabetes by pharmacological treatment of insulin resistance in high-risk Hispanic women. Diabetes 2002; 51: 2796–803.

52. Yusuf S, Gerstein H, Hoogwerf B et al. Ramipril and the development of diabetes. JAMA 2001; 286: 1882–5.

53. Saydah SH, Fradkin J, Cowie CC. Poor control of risk factors for vascular disease among adults with previously diagnosed diabetes. JAMA 2004; 291: 335–42.

54. Saaddine JB, Engelgau MM, Beckles GL et al. A diabetes report card for the United States: quality of care in the 1990s. Ann Intern Med 2002; 136: 565–74.

Chapter 2

Diabetes mellitus and schizophrenia

Oscar Villaverde

Introduction

Schizophrenia is a chronic psychiatric disorder that is characterized by abnormalities in thinking, emotions, and behavior. It usually affects 1% of the population, typically beginning before age 25 years and persisting throughout the life of the individual.[1] It is associated with significant morbidity, mortality, and compromised daily functioning. Persons with schizophrenia have lower life expectancies than the general population, primarily associated with increased risk of cardiovascular death.[2] Endocrine and cardiovascular disorders are, in fact, among the most common medical problems affecting these patients.

Numerous reports have consistently found an association between schizophrenia and diabetes. Some of the reasons that have been offered for the increased risk for type 2 diabetes mellitus (DM) in this population include a predisposition to DM, less healthy lifestyles, poorer health care, and side effects of antipsychotics.[3] Additionally, the negative symptoms and cognitive dysfunction associated with schizophrenia may further contribute to self-neglect and failure to seek treatment for medical conditions. Furthermore, the stigma associated with serious mental illness, as well as the general medical community's discomfort and fear related to working with patients who have serious mental illness, may render such patients unwelcome in medical clinics and thus influence the care they receive.[4] This chapter looks at the prevalence of glucose intolerance, DM, and diabetic ketoacidosis (DKA) in persons with schizophrenia before and after the introduction of antipsychotic medication treatment. The mechanisms by which the atypical antipsychotics may cause DM will be discussed in a later chapter. Recent literature on the contribution of exercise and nutrition programs will also be reviewed. Lastly, recommendations for the monitoring of these patients will be made.

Association between schizophrenia diagnosis and diabetes mellitus

Studies conducted before the advent of antipsychotics have suggested that schizophrenia itself may be an independent risk factor for DM.[5] For many years, schizophrenia was associated with both impaired glucose tolerance and insulin resistance. Lorenz, in 1922, reported that some of his patients with catatonic dementia praecox developed hyperglycemia in response to glucose ingestion.[6] Braceland et al, in 1945, found delayed action of insulin in patients with schizophrenia.[7] In 1946, Freeman looked at insulin response in 93 soldiers with psychiatric disorders and found that the psychiatric patients had a lower reactivity to insulin than 20 control subjects.[8] In her historical review of the association of schizophrenia and DM before the development and use of antipsychotic medications, Kohen cites several studies (Raphael and Parsons, Barrett and Serre, and Henry and Mangan) that consistently found that the glucose tolerance curves of patients with schizophrenia demonstrated diabetic characteristics.[5]

Many of these studies, however, were observational in nature and the definition of diabetes and criteria for schizophrenia used then differed somewhat from those in use today. To address this problem, Ryan and colleagues designed a study to determine whether drug-naïve, first-episode patients with schizophrenia had a higher prevalence of impaired fasting glucose tolerance or type 2 DM than a healthy volunteer group. In this cross-sectional study, fasting plasma levels of glucose, insulin, lipids, and cortisol in 26 hospitalized patients with schizophrenia were obtained. The results were then compared with the same measured levels for age- and sex-matched healthy control subjects.[9] The prevalence of impaired fasting glucose tolerance in the drug naïve, first-episode patients with schizophrenia was more than 15%. There were no cases of impaired glucose tolerance among the healthy volunteers.[9] The findings of this cross-sectional study strongly suggest that schizophrenia may be an independent risk factor for diabetes.

Table 2.1 Antipsychotic medications

Typical		Atypical
Low potency	*High potency*	
Chlorpromazine	Haloperidol	Clozapine
Thioridazine	Fluphenazine	Risperidone
Perphenazine	Thiothixene	Olanzapine
Mesoridazine	Trifluoperazine	Quetiapine
		Ziprasidone
		Aripiprazole

Association between medication treatment for schizophrenia and diabetes mellitus

Typical (first-generation or conventional) antipsychotics

The typical antipsychotic medications developed in the 1950s were the first class of agents found to be effective for the treatment of psychotic symptoms. These medications are further classified into high and low potency, based on their affinity to bind to dopamine receptors (Table 2.1). The high-potency drugs are associated with more extrapyramidal symptoms (EPS), and the low-potency agents exhibit greater anticholinergic, antihistaminic and alpha-adrenergic side effects. Soon after the introduction of chlorpromazine, a low-potency agent, a series of case reports suggested that this drug had a diabetogenic effect.[10] For example, Arneson, in 1964, reported the case of a 48-year-old patient with psychosis who developed abnormal glucose tolerance shortly after starting use of chlorpromazine.[11] Dobkin and colleagues injected healthy volunteers with chlorpromazine and found that they responded with increased blood glucose levels.[5] In fact, chlorpromazine was reportedly effective in preventing hypoglycemia in patients with malignant insulinoma.[12]

Not all medications used to treat schizophrenia, however, confer the same risk for development of glucose intolerance. Haloperidol, a high-potency conventional antipsychotic, for example, was found to have no diabetogenic effect in this population.[10] In Mukerjee et al's study, four of eight patients (50%) who had been off neuroleptic drugs for at least 1 year and were not receiving neuroleptics at the time of the study, had DM. In contrast, seven of 87 patients (12.6%) who were receiving neuroleptics had DM.[10]

The risk associated with conventional antipsychotic medication use has recently been examined in large populations of persons receiving treatment for schizophrenia.[3] Dixon et al examined the database collected by the Schizophrenia Patient Outcome Research Team (PORT), which included Medicaid and Medicare data from 1991, prior to the widespread use of atypical antipsychotics.[3] They compared prevalence rates of diabetes diagnoses in the PORT sample with that of the National Health Interview Survey (NHIS). The prevalence of diabetes in the NHIS of 1994 was 7.8% in the general adult population. In the PORT sample, with a mean age of 43 years, the rate of lifetime diabetes was 14.9% and current diabetes was 10.8%,[3] significantly higher than the rates in the general adult population. In 2002, Sernyak et al conducted a retrospective prevalence study of DM in over 38 000 patients with schizophrenia in the Veterans Health Administration of the Department of Veterans Affairs.[13] Almost 16 000 patients were prescribed a typical antipsychotic. Across all ages, almost 19% of patients who received a prescription for a typical antipsychotic medication also had a diagnosis of DM, much higher than the reported prevalence of DM in the general adult population of the USA.

Atypical (second-generation) antipsychotics

The atypical antipsychotics were introduced in the 1990s and are currently experiencing widespread use throughout the world to treat psychotic and mood disorders. These drugs are considered to be 'atypical' in that they demonstrate lower incidence rates of EPS and tardive dyskinesia (TD) than do the 'typical' drugs.[14] While first holding out promise that these medications would prove to have preferred side-effect profiles, with at least, equal antipsychotic efficacy, clinicians and researchers have come to realize that while EPS and TD do occur less frequently, these medications are now associated with other adverse effects. In particular, there has been growing concern over the metabolic side effects of excessive weight gain, glucose intolerance, new-onset type 2 DM, DKA, and dyslipidemias.

The association between atypical antipsychostic medications and glucose intolerance was first reported in patients taking clozapine. In 1998, Hagg et al compared the prevalence of glucose intolerance or diabetes in clozapine-treated patients with that of patients treated with conventional depot antipsychotics.[12] Of those patients treated with oral clozapine, 12% (7/60) had type 2 DM and 10% (6/60) had impaired glucose tolerance (IGT). By comparison, the rates for patients treated with depot antipsychotics were 6% (4/63) for type 2 DM and 3% (2/63) for IGT. This was not a prospective, study, however.

In 2000, Henderson and colleagues completed a 5-year naturalistic study of patients treated with clozapine to examine the incidence of treatment-emergent DM.[15] Surprisingly, more than one-third of the subjects (30/82) developed DM during the 60-month period. Patients experienced significant amounts of weight gain that continued to month 46; however, weight gain was not a significant risk factor for the development of DM.

Koller et al then pooled results of the Food and Drug Administration (FDA) MedWatch surveillance program with published cases of hyperglycemia associated with clozapine use. They identified 384 patients that had been placed on clozapine who developed hyperglycemia.[16] The majority, 242 patients (63%), were diagnosed with new-onset DM, and 54 patients had exacerbation of pre-existing disease. Eighty patients developed DKA and 25 patients died during hyperglycemic episodes. Forty-six patients demonstrated improved glycemic control after discontinuation or dose reduction of clozapine, further strengthening the evidence for a possible causal relationship between the medication and development of DM.

Unfortunately, the development of glucose intolerance, DM, or DKA has now also been reported with other atypical antipsychotics. In 1998, Wirshing et al reported two cases of olanzapine-associated DM.[17] Subsequently, in 2002, Koller and Doraiswamy conducted an epidemiologic survey of patients treated with olanzapine.[18] They identified 237 olanzapine-treated patients who developed hyperglycemia. Of the 237 patients, 188 (79%) were diagnosed with new-onset DM and 44 patients had exacerbation of pre-existing disease. Seventy-three percent of all cases of hyperglycemia appeared within 6 months of the start of olanzapine therapy. Eighty patients experienced metabolic acidosis or ketosis and 15 patients died. Similarly, among patients treated with risperidone, Koller et al identified 131 patients who developed hyperglycemia.[19] Of these, 78 patients (59%) had newly diagnosed hyperglycemia and 46 had exacerbation of previous DM. Twenty-six patients with acidosis or ketosis were reported and four patients died.

In 2003, Jin and colleagues analyzed 45 published cases of new-onset DM or DKA following the initiation of an atypical antipsychotic.[20] Of the 45 patients, medication treatment was as follows: 20 clozapine, 19 olanzapine, 3 quetiapine, and 3 risperidone. At baseline, 84% were over ideal body weight, but none had diabetes. The vast majority of patients, but not all, developed DM within the first 6 months of commencing atypical antipsychotic treatment (59% at 3 months and 84% at 6 months). In 32 patients with available data on follow-up weights, 50% manifested no weight gain at time of presentation with DM, suggesting that weight gain may not be the sole factor leading to DM. Importantly, 42% of these patients presented in DKA. This was alarming, as DKA is a medical emergency that typically indicates severe metabolic stress, and has associated high mortality rates. It is possible, however, that those cases that were most severe or unexpected were more likely to be reported and published.

The retrospective prevalence study of DM in veterans with schizophrenia previously described included patients who received a prescription for atypical antipsychotics.[13] Of 38 632 patients included in the study, 22 648 (58.6%) had received any atypical neuroleptic. After controlling for age, patients who received atypical antipsychotics were 9% more likely to have DM than those who received typical antipsychotics. Additionally, the prevalence of DM was significantly increased for patients who received clozapine, olanzapine, and quetiapine, but not risperidone. However, for patients < 40 years old, all of the atypical medications were associated with a significantly increased prevalence of DM. Similarly, the United Kingdom General Practice Research Database found an increased risk of DM among users of antipsychotics, with second-generation medications associated with greater risk.[21]

More recently, CATIE (Clinical Antipsychotic Trials of Intervention Effectiveness) Phase II reported that patients receiving olanzapine gained more weight than did patients taking risperidone, quetiapine or ziprasidone.[22] No patients taking ziprasidone discontinued drug due to weight gain, compared with patients taking risperidone (5%), olanzapine (8%), or quetiapine (10%). Olanzapine was also associated with substantial increases in total cholesterol and triglycerides, whereas risperidone and ziprasidone were associated with decreases in these parameters.

Association between obesity, schizophrenia, and diabetes mellitus

Obesity is defined as a body mass index (BMI) $>30\,kg/m^2$. Waist circumference, an indirect measurement of intra-abdominal fat, is another clinically important obesity-related measurement. Normal waist circumference is <40 inches in men and <35 inches in women. A high waist circumference is associated with metabolic syndrome, a precursor to the development of DM. Whereas the BMI has increased in the general population, among patients with schizophrenia, particularly women, mean BMIs are reportedly even higher.[23] Almost all available antipsychotic medications have had weight gain as a reported side effect. In a recent meta-analysis to estimate and compare the effects of antipsychotics on weight, clozapine and olanzapine were associated with the largest weight gain ($>4\,kg$), followed by chlorpromazine, sertindole, and risperidone. Weight gain with ziprasidone was insignificant ($0.04\,kg$).[24] A weight gain of $>7\%$ was reported in over half of patients treated with quetiapine in the Canadian National Outcomes Measurement Study in Schizophrenia.[25] The little that is known about aripiprazole suggests that it may have less effect on weight than other atypical antipsychotics, except ziprasidone.[26]

Factors associated with weight gain in patients taking antipsychotic medication include pretreatment BMI, length of treatment, choice of antipsychotic medication, and concomitant treatment with other medications. Weight gain may start shortly after initiation of drug treatment, but it may not plateau for more than 1 year. The addition of some mood stabilizers, particularly lithium and valproate, may increase the weight gain.

Prevention, identification, and management of diabetes mellitus in schizophrenia

Management of DM risk in persons with schizophrenia is based on addressing known risk factors. Three basic strategies can be used:

1. *Education* for the patient and his/her caregivers regarding the important role of a healthy diet, exercise, and tobacco cessation.

2. *Screening* for diabetes risk factors and early detection of metabolic syndrome in routine mental health clinical practice.
3. Development of effective *partnerships* with primary care providers to ensure access to quality medical care for patients with schizophrenia.

Healthy lifestyle choices, including diet and exercise, are the mainstay of DM prevention. All patients with schizophrenia, at a minimum, should receive education regarding healthy dietary choices and the importance of daily exercise. Structured programs that emphasize skill acquisition, social reinforcements, and incremental approaches to behavioral change are particularly effective for overweight patients with schizophrenia. For example, Menza and colleagues conducted a prospective study to look at the feasibility and efficacy of a multimodal weight control program for overweight mentally ill patients who had gained weight while taking atypical antipsychotics.[27] Thirty-one patients with schizophrenia or schizoaffective disorder participated in the 52-week program that incorporated nutrition, exercise, and behavioral interventions. Patients were encouraged to engage in light to moderate exercise through aerobic walking activities that were incorporated into group sessions. The behavioral interventions included stress management, stimulus control, self-monitoring of eating and physical activity, problem solving, and social support. In recognition of the cognitive deficits of patients with chronic mental illness, special teaching approaches were utilized, such as repetition, homework, and the use of visual materials. When compared with the non-intervention group, the intervention group experienced a mean weight loss of 6.6 lb (compared with a 7 lb gain in the non-intervention group), a significant improvement in hemoglobin A_{1c} (HbA_{1c}), and a significant decrease in blood pressure readings.

Evans and colleagues performed a randomized controlled trial that investigated the impact of individual nutrition education on weight gain in the 3 and 6 months following the start of olanzapine.[28] Fifty-one patients were randomly assigned to either an intervention or a control group. The individuals in the intervention group received six 1-hour nutrition education sessions over a 3-month period. They found that after 3 months, 64% of the control group had gained more than 7% of their initial weight, compared with only 13% of the intervention group. In addition, 22% of the intervention group actually lost weight, whereas no one in the control group lost weight.[27]

Several expert panels have made recommendations for monitoring DM risk in patients taking atypical antipsychotic medications.[29] We have adapted the recommendations to include recognition that all patients with schizophrenia are at increased risk for DM, not just those taking atypical antipsychotic medications. All patients with schizophrenia should therefore be screened for risk factors for diabetes, including a personal and family history of obesity, diabetes, dyslipidemias, hypertension, or cardiovascular disease. For women, a history of gestational diabetes should also be obtained. At this baseline visit, weight, blood pressure, and waist circumference should be measured, a BMI calculated, and a fasting glucose and lipid panel (including total, low-density lipoprotein [LDL], and high-density lipoprotein [HDL] cholesterol; and triglycerides) should also be obtained. If risk factors are thus identified, the choice of antipsychotic should be one less associated with weight gain and hyperglycemia. Patients, caregivers, and family members should also receive education about the symptoms of diabetes (polyuria, polydipsia, weight loss) and DKA (rapid onset of polydipsia, polyuria, weight loss, nausea, vomiting, dehydration, rapid respiration, confusion, drowsiness).

Weight and BMI should be reassessed at 4, 8, and 12 weeks after initiating therapy or changing medication, and quarterly thereafter. Weight gain that exceeds 5% of baseline should lead to an intervention, including patient education, a nutritional consultation, and consideration of change of medication through cross-titration. In patients for whom a switch to a different antipsychotic medication is clinically contraindicated, weight-loss pharmacotherapy may be a consideration. This would be particularly true if the BMI is $> 27 \, \text{kg/m}^2$. Sibutramine, a norepinephrine, serotonin, and dopamine receptor inhibitor may exacerbate psychotic symptoms and is contraindicated in patients with pre-existing hypertension and heart disease. Orlistat inhibits pancreatic lipase and blocks fat absorption. It is associated with gastrointestinal side effects, and may lead to fat-soluble vitamin deficiencies. Case reports have suggested that topiramate may help in weight reduction in clozapine-related weight gain.

Fasting plasma glucose, lipid levels, and blood pressure should also be assessed 3 months after initiation of therapy, and annually thereafter. Laboratory abnormalities should prompt a clinical analysis of the risks vs benefits of continuing medication treatment with the agent the patient is taking. Additionally, close communication must occur with the patient's primary care provider, in order to provide early interventions for hyperglycemia or dyslipidemias. Patients with schizophrenia who develop diabetes should have access to and receive the same quality care afforded to diabetic patients without schizophrenia. Providers must encourage them to adhere to medical treatment and visits, including annual retinal and foot sensory examinations, HbA$_{1c}$ checks, and control of blood pressure.

Conclusion

In summary, schizophrenia is associated with DM for a variety of reasons. Patients with schizophrenia are more likely than the general population to be overweight and obese, even before the age of antipsychotic treatments. The use of both typical and atypical antipsychotic medications has been associated with weight gain, glucose intolerance, and treatment-emergent DM. All patients with schizophrenia should be screened for diabetes risk factors. ADA/APA Consensus Guideline recommendations are useful in early detection of pre-diabetic and diabetic states. Recent studies have shown that patients with schizophrenia can and do respond to structured weight control and exercise programs. Close partnerships with primary care providers are invaluable in providing excellent quality care for patients with diabetes and schizophrenia.

References

1. Sadock BJ, Sadock VA, eds. Kaplan and Sadock's Synopsis of Psychiatry. Philadelphia, PA: Lippincott Williams & Wilkins, 2003.
2. Enger C, Weatherby LJ, Reynolds RF, Glasser DB, Walker AM. Serious cardiovascular events and mortality among patients with schizophrenia. J Nerv Ment Dis 2004; 192(1): 19–27.
3. Dixon L, Weiden P, Delahanty J et al. Prevalence and correlates of diabetes in national schizophrenia samples. Schizophr Bull 2000; 26: 903–12.
4. Felker B, Yazel JJ, Short D. Mortality and medical comorbidity among psychiatric patients: a review. Psychiatr Serv 1996; 47: 1356–63.
5. Kohen D. Diabetes mellitus and schizophrenia: historical perspective. Br J Psychiatry 2004; Suppl 47: S64–6.
6. Lorenz WF. Sugar tolerance in dementia praecox and other mental disorders. Arch Neurol Psychiatry 1922; 8: 184–96.
7. Braceland FJ, Meduna LJ, Vaichulis JA. Delayed action of insulin in schizophrenia. Am J Psychiatry 1945; 102: 108–10.

8. Freeman H. Resistance to insulin in mentally disturbed soldiers. Arch Neurol Psychiatry 1946; 56: 74–8.

9. Ryan MC, Collins P, Thakore JH. Impaired fasting glucose tolerance in first-episode, drug-naive patients with schizophrenia. Am J Psychiatry 2003; 160: 284–9.

10. Mukherjee S, Decina P, Bocola V et al. Diabetes mellitus in schizophrenic patients. Compr Psychiatry 1996; 37: 68–73.

11. Arneson GA. Phenothiazine derivatives and glucose metabolism. J Neuropsychiatry 1964; 5: 181–5.

12. Hagg S, Joelsson L, Mjornadal T et al. Prevalence of diabetes and impaired glucose tolerance in patients with clozapine compared with patients treated with conventional depot neuroleptic medications. J Clin Psychiatry 1998; 59: 294–9.

13. Sernyak MJ, Leslie DL, Alarcon RD. Association of diabetes mellitus with use of atypical neuroleptics in the treatment of schizophrenia. Am J Psychiatry 2004; 159: 561–6.

14. Jin H, Meyer JM, Jeste DV. Atypical antipsychotics and glucose dysregulation: a systematic review. Schizophr Res 2004; 71: 195–212.

15. Henderson DC, Cagliero E, Gray C et al. Clozapine, diabetes mellitus, weight gain, and lipid abnormalities: a five-year naturalistic study. Am J Psychiatry 2000; 157: 975–81.

16. Koller E, Schneider B, Bennett K et al. Clozapine-associated diabetes. Am J Med 2001; 111: 716–23.

17. Wirshing DA, Spellberg BJ, Erhart SM, Marder SR, Wirshing WC. Novel antipsychotics and new onset diabetes. Biol Psychiatry 1998; 44: 778–83.

18. Koller EA, Doraiswamy PM. Olanzapine-associated diabetes mellitus. Pharmacotherapy 2002; 22: 841–52.

19. Koller E, Cross JT, Doraiswamy PM, Schneider BS. Risperidone-associated diabetes mellitus: a pharmacovigilance study. Pharmacotherapy 2003; 23: 735–44.

20. Jin H, Meyer JM, Jeste DV. Phenomenology of and risk factors for new-onset diabetes mellitus and diabetic ketoacidosis associated with atypical antipsychotics: an analysis of 45 published cases. Ann Clin Psychiatry 2002; 14: 59–64.

21. Kornegay CJ, Vasilakis-Scaramozza C, Jick H. Incident diabetes associated with antipsychotic use in the United Kingdom general practice research database. J Clin Psychiatry 2002; 63(9): 758–62.

22. Stroup TS, Lieberman JA, McEvoy et al. Effectiveness of olanzapine, quetiapine, risperidone, and ziprasidone in patients with chronic schizophrenia following discontinuation of a previous atypical antipsychotic. Am J Psychiatry 2006; 163: 611–22.

23. Homel P, Casey D, Allison DB. Changes in BMI for individuals with and without schizophrenia, 1987–1996. Schizophr Res 2002; 55(3): 277–84.

24. Allison DB, Mentore JL, Heo M et al. Antipsychotic-induced weight gain: a comprehensive research synthesis. Am J Psychiatry 1999; 156(11): 1686–96.

25. McIntyre RS, Trakas K, Lin D et al. Risk of weight gain associated with antipsychotic treatment: results from the Canadian National Outcomes Measurement Study in Schizophrenia. Can J Psychiatry 2003; 48(10): 689–94.

26. American Diabetes Association, American Psychiatric Association, American Association of Clinical Endocrinologists, North American Association for the Study of Obesity. Consensus development conference on antipsychotic drugs and obesity and diabetes. Diabetes Care 2004; 27(2): 596–601.

27. Menza M, Vreeland B, Minsky S et al. Managing atypical antipsychotic-associated weight gain: 12-month data on a multimodal weight control program. J Clin Psychiatry 2004; 65: 471–7.
28. Evans S, Newton R, Higgins S. Nutritional intervention to prevent weight gain in patients commenced on olanzapine: a randomized controlled trial. Aust N Z J Psychiatry 2005; 39: 479–86.
29. Marder SR, Essock SM, Miller AL et al. Physical health monitoring of patients with schizophrenia. Am J Psychiatry 2004; 161(8): 1334–49.

Chapter 3

Diabetes mellitus and depression

Julie E Malphurs

Introduction

Approximately 16% of the population will suffer from depression at any time during their lifetime.[1] This lifetime prevalence will increase significantly with age, as well as with the existence of a co-occurring physical condition. The number of US citizens with diagnosed diabetes is projected to increase 165% from 11 million in 2000 to 29 million in 2050, with the largest percent increase occurring among those persons ≥75 years old (+271% in older women; +437% in older men).[2]

Depressive symptoms have an adverse impact on symptom burden, functional impairment, adherence to medication regimens, and self-management of illness.[3,4] Persons with co-occurring medical diseases such as diabetes or cardiovascular conditions have a significantly higher risk of complications, including mortality, than persons with no depressive symptoms.[5-7] Persons with diabetes and depressive symptoms have mortality rates nearly twice as high as persons with diabetes and no depressive symptomatology.[8] Persons with co-occurring medical illness and depression also have higher health care utilization, leading to higher direct and indirect health care costs[9,10] and it has been suggested that co-occurring medical illness and depression may be key barriers to achieving treatment goals.[11] It is thus important to understand the relationship between co-occurring mental and physical disorders because of their potential for modifying patient outcomes. One of the current priority research areas of the National Institute of Mental Health is to decrease the impact of depression on co-occurring illnesses, specifically diabetes and cardiovascular disease.[12]

Costs

Persons with both diabetes and depression have total health care expenditures nearly 5 times higher than diabetic persons without depression, nearly US$195 billion.[13,14] The increase in total health care expenditures is largely the result of increased medical rather than mental health utilization and has also been shown to occur in a relatively short amount of time (6 months).[13,15] The higher health care utilization and expenditures among persons with diabetes and depression remain even after controlling for age, gender, ethnicity, and other co-occurring medical conditions.[13,16] Furthermore, older adults with diabetes and depression have 21% greater annual non-mental health-related expenditures and 85% greater annual Medicare payments than older adults with diabetes only.[15,17]

Depression and diabetes – overview

Persons with diabetes are twice as likely to have depression as non-diabetic persons.[18] A review of 20 studies on the comorbidity of depression and diabetes found that the average prevalence was about 15%, and ranged from 8.5 to 40%, three times the rate of depressive disorders found in the general adult population of the USA.[18–20] The rates of clinically significant depressive symptoms among persons with diabetes are even higher – ranging from 21.8% to 60.0%.[21] Recent studies have indicated that persons with type II diabetes, accompanied by either major or minor depression, have significantly higher mortality rates than non-depressed persons with diabetes.[8] Links have also been established between depression, diabetes, and an increased risk of cardiovascular and cerebrovascular complications.[8] Older adults with diabetes mellitus (DM) are significantly more likely to develop major depression than other older adults, and older Latinos with diabetes have the highest reported rates of depression.[17,22,23]

Etiology

Depression has important clinical relevance to DM due to its potential association with poor glycemic control and decreased adherence to treatment regimens. However, it is still unclear what the etiology is behind the strong association between these two illnesses. There are several possible mechanisms to explain the relationship between depressive symptoms and DM, and none have been absolutely supported by an evidence base to date.

One view is that the depressive symptoms are triggered by the existence of DM. Depressive symptoms are associated with biochemical changes related to the DM (i.e. hyperglycemia, inflammation, activation of the hypothalamic–pituitary–adrenal axis [HPA], stress) and may be important factors in disrupting overall metabolic control.[20,24,25] Further, the presence of depression and depressive symptoms may present as a result of lifestyle choices (i.e. poor diet, no physical activity) that are frequently associated with the presence of DM.

An alternative explanation for the relationship between depression and DM views the development of DM as the result of pre-existing depression. This view suggests that:

- neurohormonal changes induced by depression, such as hypercortisolism, can lead to insulin resistance and to the development of DM
- behavioral factors associated with depression, including lack of physical activity and poor diet, increase the risk for the development of DM.[22,26]

The presence of depression may adversely impact the function of a number of neurotransmitters, including serotonin, norepinephrine, dopamine, acetylcholine, and γ-aminobutyric acid and (GABA).[20] In addition, depression can cause abnormalities in the HPA axis and other hormonal irregularities. Meta-analyses have determined an association between depression and hyperglycemia, but the mechanism and directionality of the association has not been determined.[20,27] The increase in glycosylated hemoglobin (HbA_{1c}) levels attributed to depression alone has ranged from 1.8 to 3.3%.[27,28] A meta-analysis of depression and studies of glycemic control confirmed the association of depression with hyperglycemia, but was unable to reveal the mechanism or the direction of the association.[27] The association between depression and glycemic control has recently been observed in ethnic minority groups with diabetes as well.[29] In addition, treatment and subsequent improvement in depression has been significantly associated with improvement in glycemic control.

It is extremely difficult to establish an evidence base for either of these explanations, because of the lack of control populations and standardized measurements. The role of stress in the development of depression as well as glucose regulation has been well-established, and the impact of stress can be nearly impossible to disentangle in studies of DM and depression. While the relationship between DM and depression clearly exists, the causative nature of this relationship may always be difficult to determine due to the circular directionality of these two illnesses. Depression may be a cause or a result of diabetes, and both the direction and the mechanism of this relationship may vary over time. Regardless of the etiology of these illnesses in a patient, the outcomes for both illnesses worsen when they co-occur, than with either illness alone.

Diabetes mellitus and depression – outcomes and symptoms

DM, similar to depression, is a chronic illness that can impact multiple physical and physiological systems in the body. Physical symptoms are often assumed to be related to diabetes with little to no consideration given to the potential impact of co-occurring mood or other psychological conditions. DM symptoms may, in fact, be unreliable indicators of poor glycemic control when symptoms of depression are present in an individual. A study of typical DM-related symptoms was conducted and found that depression, not DM (glycemic control), was the better predictor of most DM-related symptoms when both DM and depression are present (Table 3.1).[30]

A meta-analysis of the relationship between depression and DM complications (types I and II) indicated that an increase in the number of depressive symptoms is associated with an increase in the severity and number of DM complications, including retinopathy, neuropathy, and nephropathy.[31] Table 3.2 indicates symptom criteria for major depression. It should be noted that dysthymia and other disorders of mood may not meet criteria for depression but result in symptomatology that have a significant impact on functioning. At a minimum, all patients with diabetes should be screened annually for depressive symptoms. A simple two-question patient self-administered screen

Table 3.1   Correlations of diabetes mellitus symptoms with depression scores and glycosylated hemoglobin (HbA_{1c}).[30]

Symptom	Depression+[a]	HbA_{1c}
Hyperglycemic symptoms		
Thirst	0.41[b]	0.18
Frequent urination	0.46[b]	0.22
Losing weight	0.18	0.00
Hypoglycemic symptoms		
Hunger	0.31[b]	0.14
Sweating	0.37[b]	0.04
Trembling	0.47[b]	0.12
Fainting/dizziness	0.25[b]	0.11
Loss of consciousness	0.08	0.26[b]
Non-specific symptoms		
Fatigue	0.65[b]	0.11
Fever, feeling ill	0.48[b]	0.13

[a]Positive depression score as indicated on the Beck Depression Inventory.

[b]Indicates $p<0.05$, all statistically significant correlations remained significant in a multiple regression analysis when depression and glucose control were examined together, with the exception of loss of consciousness.

(Table 3.3) is clinically effective in easily identifying many of these patients.

Compared to persons with either DM or depression, individuals with co-occurring DM and depression have shown poorer adherence to dietary and physical activity recommendations, decreased adherence to hypoglycemic medication regimens, higher health care costs, increases in HbA_{1c} levels, poorer glycemic control, higher rates of retinopathy and macrovascular complications such as stroke and myocardial infarction, and higher ambulatory care use and use of prescriptions.[11,13,34–37] DM and depressive symptoms have been shown to have strong independent effects on physical functioning, and individuals experiencing either of these conditions will have worse functional outcomes than those with neither or only one condition.[34,35]

Age-related impairments and physical changes may also complicate the ability to self-manage a chronic illness. Nearly all of DM management is conducted by the patient, and those with co-occurring depression may have poorer outcomes and increased risk of complications due to poorer adherence to glucose, diet, and medication

Table 3.2 DSM-IV criteria for major depression

A. Five (or more) of the following symptoms have been present during the same 2-week period and represent a change from previous functioning; at least one of the symptoms is either: (1) depressed mood or (2) loss of interest or pleasure.

Note: Do not include symptoms that are clearly due to a general medical condition, or mood-incongruent delusions or hallucinations.

(1) depressed mood most of the day, nearly every day, as indicated by either subjective report (e.g. feels sad or empty) or observation made by others (e.g. appears tearful)
Note: In children and adolescents, can be irritable mood.

(2) markedly diminished interest or pleasure in all, or almost all, activities most of the day, nearly every day (as indicated by either subjective account or observation made by others)

(3) significant weight loss when not dieting or weight gain (e.g. a change of more than 5% of body weight in a month), or decrease or increase in appetite nearly every day
Note: In children, consider failure to make expected weight gains.

(4) insomnia or hypersomnia nearly every day

(5) psychomotor agitation or retardation nearly every day (observable by others, not merely subjective feelings of restlessness or being slowed down)

(6) fatigue or loss of energy nearly every day

(7) feelings of worthlessness or excessive or inappropriate guilt (which may be delusional) nearly every day (not merely self-reproach or guilt about being sick)

(8) diminished ability to think or concentrate, or indecisiveness, nearly every day (either by subjective account or as observed by others)

(9) recurrent thoughts of death (not just fear of dying), recurrent suicidal ideation without a specific plan, or a suicide attempt or a specific plan for committing suicide

Reproduced from *Diagnostic and Statistical Manual of Mental Disorders*, 4th edn.[32] with permission.

Table 3.3 Two-question screen for depression[33]

1. During the past month, have you often been bothered by feeling down, depressed, or hopeless?
2. During the past month, have you often been bothered by little interest or pleasure in doing things?

regimens.[27,34,36] The lowest adherence to dietary and exercise recommendations is among older adults with the highest levels of depressive symptom severity.[26,36] Increasing physical activity has been shown to improve both DM and depression outcomes[26,38] and a program promoting walking is safe for most patients, including many older adults with medical illness.[11,38,39] There is some evidence that treatment of depression with antidepressant and/or cognitive-behavioral therapies can improve glycemic control and glucose regulation without any change in the treatment for DM.

Treatment

Despite the lack of a definitive cause–effect model to explain the significant relationship between depression and DM, reports on the effects of treatment for depression have shown promise on outcomes for both diseases. Treatment for depression in patients with DM has demonstrated benefits on glycemic control as well as mood, and even insulin sensitivity.[24,40] There is evidence that both antidepressant medication and psychotherapeutic treatments can improve both depressive and DM outcomes in patients with both illnesses. Recently, collaborative care models in primary care using case management interventions for the treatment of depression have shown promise in improving outcomes in patients with DM.[41,42]

Antidepressant medications

Antidepressant therapy has shown a positive impact on both mood and glucose regulation in individuals with DM and depression.[27,43–46] In a limited open-label study of sertraline, patients with DM (HbA_{1c} >8) and depressive symptoms, based on Hamilton Depression Scale (HAM-D) ratings, showed decreases in HAM-D scores and a statistically significant decrease in HbA_{1c} from an average 9.2 to 8.8.[45] Several studies of fluoxetine in patients with DM and depression have indicated reductions in weight and in HbA_{1c} to near-normal levels (<7).[46] A double-blind placebo-controlled study of nortriptyline showed considerable effect on depressive symptomatology while at the same time indicating significant improvement in glucose control in patients with DM and depression.[43] Side effects of frequently used antidepressants should be considered, especially when used in an older population. Table 3.4 indicates common side effects of antidepressant medications that are of particular relevance in a DM population.

More double-blind, controlled studies of antidepressant treatments need to be conducted on larger populations of patients with DM and depression in order to obtain an evidence base with which to establish treatment guidelines for use. Currently, the evidence suggests that treatment of depression improves both depressive symptoms as well as DM symptoms at clinically, if not statistically, significant levels.

Psychotherapy

In addition to pharmacological treatments for depression, current research has also indicated benefits from psychological therapies. The introduction or inclusion of various types of behavioral interventions in the management of DM has been demonstrated to improve metabolic control as well as quality of life. To date, however, there has been little empirical support for the successful use of non-pharmacological therapies (i.e. psychotherapies) for the management of depression specifically in persons with DM. Non-pharmacological interventions are particularly useful in the initial management of patients who may have mild depressive symptoms and are concerned about taking medications.

Other forms of psychotherapy, specifically cognitive-behavioral psychotherapy have been shown useful in the treatment of depression in persons with DM. Cognitive-behavioral therapy (CBT) is characterized by implementing behavioral strategies to engage patients in social and physical activities as well as employing problem-solving and cognitive methods to identify and replace maladaptive thought patterns with more adaptive and useful thoughts. Lustman and colleagues[47] performed a randomized, controlled investigation of the use of CBT for depression in patients with type II DM. CBT was found to be an effective treatment for depression and also led to a significant decrease in HbA_{1c} levels compared with the control group. Collaborative care models have used case management, in conjunction with problem-solving therapy, for the treatment of depression in DM populations.[48] Future investigations of non-pharmacological interventions may yield similar results and provide alternative and adjunctive methods for treatment of depression in patients with DM as well as other chronic medical conditions.

Table 3.4   Common side effects of antidepressant medications with relevance to diabetes mellitus

Medication	Side effect		
	Sedation	Cardiovascular	Weight gain
Tricyclic agents[a]	×	×	×
MAO inhibitors[b]	×	×	×
Benzodiazepines[c]	×		
SSRIs[d]	×		+/−

[a]Tricyclic antidepressant treatment may also be a useful therapy for diabetic neuropathy.
[b]MAO inhibitors, monoamine oxidase inhibitors.
[c]Benzodiazepines are not a recommended first-line treatment for depression.
[d]SSRIs, selective serotonin reuptake inhibitors: sertraline and fluoxetine.

Conclusions

Clinicians treating DM patients must have a high index of suspicion regarding the possible presence of depressive symptoms and/or major depressive disorder. All patients with diabetes, at a minimum, should be screened for depressive symptoms on an annual basis. The main clinical aim is to identify and treat these depressive symptoms. Providing this service to patients not only alleviates depressive symptoms but also has a significant impact on improving mental and physical functioning, adherence with disease self-management and medication regimens, and diabetes outcomes, including HbA_{1c} levels.

References

1. Kessler RC, Berglund P, Demler O et al. The epidemiology of major depressive disorder: results from the National Comorbidity Survey Replication. JAMA 2003; 289: 3095–105.
2. Boyle JP, Honeycutt AA, Narayan V et al. Projection of diabetes burden through 2050: impact of changing demography and disease prevalence in the United States. Diabetes Care 2001; 24: 1936–40.
3. Wells KB, Stewart A, Hays RD et al. The functioning and well-being of depressed patients: results from the medical outcomes study. JAMA 1989; 262: 914–19.
4. Lyness JM, Bruce ML, Koenig HG et al. Depression and medical illness in late life: report of a symposium. J Am Geriatr Soc 1996; 44: 198–203.

5. Gallo JJ, Bogner HR, Morales KH et al. Depression, cardiovascular disease, diabetes, and two-year mortality among older, primary-care patients. Am J Geriatr Psychiatry 2005; 13: 748–55.
6. Pennix BW, Geerlings SW, Deeg DJ et al. Minor and major depression and the risk of death in older persons. Arch Gen Psychiatry 1999; 56: 889–95.
7. Schulz R, Beach SR, Ives DG et al. Association between depression and mortality in older adults: the Cardiovascular Health Study. Arch Intern Med 2000; 160: 1761–8.
8. Katon WJ, Rutter C, Simon G et al. The association of comorbid depression with mortality in patients with type 2 diabetes. Diabetes Care 2005; 28: 2668–72.
9. Simon GE, Von Korff M, Barlow W. Health care costs of primary care patients with recognized depression. Arch Gen Psychiatry 1995; 52: 850–6.
10. Unutzer J, Patrick DL, Simon G et al. Depressive symptoms and the cost of health services in HMO patients aged 65 years and older: a four-year prospective study. JAMA 1997; 277: 1618–23.
11. Piette JD, Richardson C, Valenstein M. Addressing the needs of patients with multiple chronic illnesses: the case of diabetes and depression. Am J Manag Care 2004; 10 (Part 2): 152–62.
12. Insel TR, Charney DS. Research on major depression: strategies and priorities. JAMA 2003; 289: 3167–8.
13. Egede LE, Zheng D, Simpson K. Comorbid depression is associated with increased health care use and expenditures in individuals with diabetes. Diabetes Care 2002; 25: 464–70.
14. Simon GE, Katon WJ, Lin EH et al. Diabetes complications and depression as predictors of health service costs. Gen Hosp Psychiatry 2005: 27: 344–51.
15. Finkelstein EA, Bray JW, Chen H et al. Prevalence and costs of major depression among elderly claimants with diabetes. Diabetes Care 2003; 26: 415–20.
16. Hodgson TA, Cohen AJ. Medical care expenditures for diabetes, its chronic complications and its comorbidities. Prev Med 1999; 29: 173–86.
17. California Healthcare Foundation & American Geriatrics Society. Guidelines for improving the care of the older person with diabetes mellitus. J Am Geriatr Soc 2003; S265–S280.
18. Anderson RJ, Freedland KE, Clouse RE et al. The prevalence of comorbid depression in adults with diabetes. Diabetes Care 2004; 24: 1069–78.
19. Gavard JA, Lustman PJ, Clouse RE. Prevalence of depression in adults with diabetes: an epidemiological evaluation. Diabetes Care 1993; 16: 1167–78.
20. Harris MD. Psychosocial aspects of diabetes with an emphasis on depression. Curr Diab Rep 2003; 3: 49–55.
21. Lustman PJ, Gavard JA. Psychosocial aspects of diabetes in adult populations. In: National Diabetes Data Group. Diabetes in America, 2nd edn. NIH Publication #95-1468, 1995.
22. Fisher L, Chesla CA, Mullan JT, Skaff MM, Kanter RA. Contributors to depression in Latino and European-American patients with type 2 diabetes. Diabetes Care 2001; 24: 1751–7.
23. Black SA, Markides KS, Ray LA. Depression predicts increased incidence of adverse health outcomes in older Mexican-Americans with type 2 diabetes. Diabetes Care 2003; 26: 2822–8.
24. Carnethon MR, Kinder LS, Fair JM, Stafford RS, Fortmann SP. Symptoms of depression as a risk factor for incident diabetes: findings from the National Health and Nutrition Examination Epidemiologic Follow-up Study, 1971–1992. Am J Epidemiol 2003; 158: 416–23.

25. Kaholokula JK, Haynes SN, Grandinetti A, Chang HK. Biological, psychosocial and sociodemographic variables associated with depressive symptoms in persons with type 2 diabetes. J Behav Med 2003; 26: 435–58.

26. Saydah SH, Brancati FL, Golden SH, Fradkin J, Harris MI. Depressive symptoms and the risk of type 2 diabetes mellitus in a US sample. Diabetes Metabol Res Rev 2003; 19: 202–8.

27. Lustman PJ, Anderson RJ, Freedland KE et al. Depression and poor glycemic control: a meta-analytic review of the literature. Diabetes Care 2000; 23: 934–42.

28. Van Tilburg M, McCaskill CC, Lane JD. Depressed mood is a factor in glycemic control in type 1 diabetes. Psychosom Med 2001; 63: 551–5.

29. Gross R, Olfson M, Gameroff MJ et al. Depression and glycemic control in Hispanic primary care patients with diabetes. J Gen Intern Med 2005; 20: 460–6.

30. Lustman PJ, Clouse RE, Carney RM. Depression and the reporting of diabetes symptoms. Int J Psychiatry Med 1988; 18: 295–303.

31. de Groot M, Anderson R, Freedland KE. Association of depression and diabetes complications: a meta-analysis. Psychosom Med 2001; 63: 619–30.

32. Diagnostic and Statistical Manual of Mental Disorders, 4th edn. American Psychiatric Association, 1994.

33. Spitzer RL, Kroenke K, Williams JBW. Validation and utility of a self-report version of the PRIME-MD: the PHQ primary care study. Primary Care Evaluation of Mental Disorders. Patient Health Questionnaire. JAMA 1999; 282: 1737–44.

34. Ciechanowski PS, Katon WJ, Russo JE et al. The relationship of depressive symptoms to symptom reporting, self-care and glucose control in diabetes. Gen Hosp Psychiatry 2003; 25: 246–52.

35. Fultz NH, Ofstedal MB, Herzog AR, Wallace RB. Additive and interactive effects of comorbid physical and mental conditions on functional health. J Aging Health 2003; 15: 465–81.

36. Ciechanowski PS, Katon WJ, Russo JE. Depression and diabetes: impact of depressive symptoms on adherence, function and costs. Arch Int Med 2000; 160: 3278–85.

37. Lustman PJ, Clouse RE. Depression in diabetic patients: the relationship between mood and glycemic control. J Diabetes Complications 2005; 19: 113–22.

38. Strawbridge WJ, Deleger S, Roberts RE et al. Physical activity reduces the risk of subsequent depression for older adults. Am J Epidemiol 2002; 156: 328–34.

39. Hu FB. Walking: the best medicine for diabetes? Arch Int Med 2003; 163: 1397–8.

40. Lustman PJ, Clouse RE. Treatment of depression in diabetes: impact on mood and medical outcome. J Psychosom Res 2002; 53: 917–24.

41. Katon WJ, Von Korff M, Lin EH et al. The Pathways Study: a randomized trial of collaborative care in patients with diabetes and depression. Arch Gen Psychiatry 2004; 61: 1042–9.

42. Williams J Jr, Katon W, Lin E et al. Effectiveness of depression care management for older adults with coexisting depression and diabetes mellitus. Ann Intern Med 2004; 140: 1015–24.

43. Lustman PJ, Griffith LS, Clouse RE et al. Effects of nortriptyline on depression and glycemic control in diabetes: results of a double-blind, placebo-controlled trial. Psychosom Med 1997; 59: 241–50.

44. Lustman PJ, Freedland KE, Griffith LS et al. Fluoxetine for depression in diabetes: a randomized double-blind placebo-controlled trial. Diabetes Care 2000; 23: 618–23.

45. Goodnick PJ, Kumar A, Henry JH et al. Sertraline in coexisting major depression and diabetes mellitus. Psychopharmacol Bull 1997; 33: 261–4.

46. Goodnick PJ. Use of antidepressants in treatment of comorbid diabetes mellitus and depression as well as in diabetic neuropathy. Ann Clin Psychiatry 2001; 13: 31–41.
47. Lustman PJ, Griffith LS, Freedland KE et al. Cognitive behavior therapy for depression in type 2 diabetes mellitus. A randomized, controlled trial. Ann Intern Med 1998; 129: 613–21.
48. Tuckington RW. Depression masquerading as diabetic neuropathy. JAMA 1980; 243: 1147–50.

Chapter 4

Diabetes mellitus and cognitive impairment

José A Luchsinger and Hermes Florez

Introduction

This chapter summarizes the evidence relating diabetes mellitus (DM) to cognitive impairment. A Medline search was conducted relating the term 'diabetes' to 'cognition', 'cognitive impairment', and 'dementia' from which most of the articles cited in this chapter were chosen. In addition, pertinent articles related to cognitive impairment were chosen by the authors. Longitudinal studies and clinical trials were favored over other types of studies when available.

Epidemiology of dementia, cognitive impairment, and diabetes mellitus

Cognitive impairment is most prevalent in the elderly. The prevalence of dementia is about 1%, beginning at age 60 years old, but can be as high as 50% in those aged ≥85 years old.[1] It is expected that this prevalence will increase with greater life expectancy and growth in the elderly population. The most important form of diabetes in adults and in the elderly is type 2 DM. Thus, this chapter will focus on the evidence relating type 2 DM to cognitive impairment and will not cover the cognitive complications of type 1 DM. According to data from the third National Nutrition and Health Examination Survey (NHANES III), the prevalence of diabetes is over 12% in persons aged ≥60 years old in the USA;[2] this prevalence is twice as high in African-Americans and Hispanics,[3] and is expected to increase. Over 50% of persons in this age group have either diabetes or glucose intolerance (at risk for diabetes) in the USA.[2] These facts underscore the potential growing importance of diabetes as a risk factor for cognitive impairment. Currently, there are no confirmed preventive or curative measures for dementia. However, one of the implications of linking diabetes to cognitive impairment is that preventing or treating diabetes may reduce the risk of cognitive impairment.

Types of cognitive impairment and scope of the problem

Cognitive impairment is a growing concern in aging societies. Several types of cognitive impairment have been described in research and clinical practice. Dementia, the most severe type and most frequently studied, is defined as cognitive impairment in several domains, usually including memory, accompanied also by functional impairment (inability to perform independently in activities of daily living). The most frequent form of dementia is Alzheimer's disease (AD),[4] which constitutes about 70% of cases. AD is usually identified clinically by short-term memory impairment of slow onset and progression, affecting other cognitive domains (e.g. attention and language), with disease progression, and ultimately causing functional impairment. The second most frequent form is vascular dementia (VD), which has usually been defined as dementia occurring within a short time of a stroke.[4] Memory may be affected in VD, but the main affected cognitive domains are related to executive frontal abilities. In many cases the temporal relationship between dementia onset and the onset of overt stroke or subclinical cerebrovascular disease (not suspected clinically, but seen in brain imaging as infarcts or white matter hyperintensities) is unclear. There is some uncertainty on whether VD and AD with a cerebrovascular component can be differentiated, and studies vary in the proportion of cases of dementia identified as VD or AD. The occurrence of clinical features of both AD and VD is often called 'mixed dementia'.

Recently, there has been a growing interest in cognitive impairment in the absence of significant functional impairment (without dementia). Two terms have been coined to describe this type of cognitive impairment: mild cognitive impairment (MCI) and cognitive impairment – no dementia (CIND). MCI is defined as the presence of memory complaints, detectable memory impairment on neuropsychological tests that is beyond 1.5 SD of the norms, and the absence of functional impairment.[5] Most persons with MCI go on to develop AD within 10 years.[6] Thus, MCI has become an area of great interest for interventions intended to prevent or slow progression to AD. There are efforts to expand the use of MCI beyond the memory domain to others such as the so-called executive frontal abilities.[6] CIND can be defined as the presence of cognitive impairment in the absence of functional impairment.[7] Lastly, cognitive impairment can be defined by performance in global measures such as the Mini-Mental State Examination (MMSE),[8] or by studying specific cognitive domains.

The most frequently studied domains in adults and the elderly are memory and executive frontal abilities. For the purpose of this chapter we will refer to conscious (explicit) memory. Memory is the ability to recall an experience after it has been extinguished.[9] Memory problems are probably the most frequent cognitive complaint that brings patients to medical attention. There are several key processes involved in the long-term maintenance of memories. One is consolidation, based in the hippocampal formation, which enables the laying down of new memories.[9] This is the process first and most prominently affected in AD and amnestic MCI, and tested in clinical practice with verbal learning tests, such as the 5-minute recall of three items of the MMSE. Another key memory process is retrieval,[9] which is most affected by lesions involving the frontal lobe subcortical circuits. Pure problems with this process imply an inability to retrieve memory from its long-term storage sites (associational cortices) in the absence of problems in consolidation. This process is commonly affected by cerebrovascular disease, and manifests by difficulty in recalling words or objects which can be aided by giving multiple choice options or cues (recognition). A person with abnormal consolidation will not be able to recognize the three recall items from the MMSE even when given cues or multiple choices, and may confabulate, whereas the person with normal consolidation but abnormal retrieval will have difficulty remembering the words, but will recognize them from a list once a cue is given.

Executive frontal abilities are those skills that are used to plan and execute complex tasks and comprise different processes such as attention, working memory, and impulse control. Executive frontal abilities are most often affected by lesions that disrupt the frontal subcortical networks,[10] the same system that supports memory retrieval. Tests of executive function commonly used in clinical practice include digits forward and backwards (working memory) and the attention items of the MMSE.

The natural history of cognitive impairment could be described as onset of cognitive impairment in some cognitive domain, which may worsen over time, present clinically as CIND or MCI, and eventually progress to dementia when the ability to live independently is impaired. In the case of AD, this usually presents as impairment in recall with memory complaints that worsen progressively, may eventually be identified as MCI or CIND, and subsequently progresses to full-blown dementia. In the case of a large or strategic stroke, dementia onset occurs abruptly within a short time of stroke, with or without preceding cognitive impairment. There is growing interest in other forms of vascular cognitive impairment, which may present slowly and incrementally with worsening 'subclinical' cerebrovascular disease (white matter hyperintensities and 'silent infarcts'), affect executive abilities and memory retrieval, and may or may not progress to the syndrome of dementia. Some consider that the cognition field has paid more attention to AD to the detriment of the identification of the other forms of cognitive impairment described here, particularly those related to executive abilities.[11] In the following paragraphs we will review evidence linking DM to the cognitive processes and syndromes described above.

Potential mechanisms linking diabetes mellitus to cognitive impairment

There are several mechanisms potentially linking DM to cognitive impairment (Figure 4.1). First, DM is a risk factor for cerebrovascular disease.[12] Thus, it is expected that DM can cause the vascular forms of cognitive impairment described previously. DM may also increase the risk of cognitive impairment through associated cardiovascular risk factors, such as hypertension and dyslipidemia, which are related primarily with an increased risk of cerebrovascular disease.[1] Secondly, DM may increase the risk of cognitive impairment processes that affect the deposition of amyloid beta (Aβ) in the brain, the putative culprit in the pathogenesis of AD.[4] Processes potentially linking DM to this mechanism include increased oxidative stress[13] and the production of

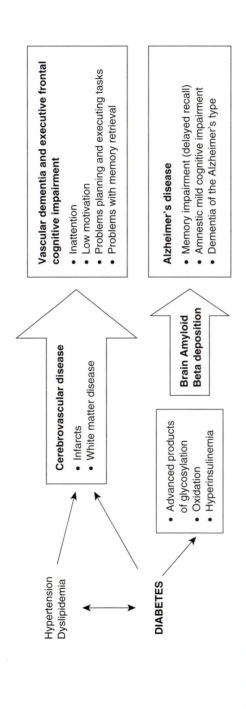

Figure 4.1 Summary of the mechanisms linking type 2 diabetes mellitus to the most often recognized forms of cognitive impairment, vascular dementia and executive frontal cognitive impairment, and Alzheimer's disease.

advanced glycation end-products (AGEs).[14] Glycation of Aβ increases its aggregation in vivo, and the participation of a receptor for AGE (RAGE) in AD has been confirmed in animal models. Moreover, antibodies against specific AGEs decrease their toxicity in cultured cells and AGEs have been proposed as biomarkers of AD risk.[14] Thirdly, hyperinsuline-mia is an important feature preceding and accompanying type 2 DM, and the role of insulin in AD has attracted increasing attention.[15] Insulin, which can cross the blood–brain barrier from the periphery to the brain, competes with Aβ for insulin degrading enzyme (IDE) in the brain, including the hippocampus.[16] This impairs the clearance of Aβ in the brain, potentially increasing its deleterious effect in AD. Manipulation of insulin levels has been demonstrated to affect cognition and levels of Aβ in the cerebrospinal fluid,[17,18] thus supporting the strong plausibility of DM as risk factor for AD. Finally, there is evidence linking DM to the presence of amyloid plaques and neurofibrillary tangles, the pathologic hallmarks of AD which has been supported by some but not all studies.[19,20]

Diabetes mellitus and risk of dementia

DM has been found consistently to be related to VD, but its relation to AD is less clear. A study of Japanese subjects aged ≥65 years old found that DM was related to a higher risk of AD (relative risk [RR] = 2.2) and VD (RR = 2.8).[21] A longitudinal study from the Netherlands in over 5000 subjects aged ≥55 years old without dementia at baseline found an RR for AD of 1.9.[22] This association was stronger in subjects with DM who reported insulin treatment. Another European study found that the risk of all-cause dementia was increased by DM (RR = 2.6), but this relation was weaker with AD (RR = 1.4).[23] A study from Rochester, Minnesota found an RR of 2 relating DM and AD,[24] similar to the study from the Netherlands. A study of Catholic nuns, priests, and brothers ≥55 years old found that DM was associated with a higher risk of AD (RR = 1.7).[25] The Honolulu–Asia Aging Study also found that DM in old age was related to a higher risk of AD (RR = 1.8) and AD pathology on autopsy, particularly in subjects with the *APOE-ε4* allele,[26] the only known genetic risk factor for sporadic AD.[4] One study from Canada found that DM had a weak non-statistically significant relation to AD (RR = 1.3), but was related to VD (RR = 2.0). A Swedish study found a similar non-significant relation to AD (RR = 1.3), and a significant relation to a higher risk of VD (RR = 2.6).[27] A prospective study in over 1000 subjects from New York City who were mostly African-American and Caribbean-Hispanic, with a mean age of 75 years, and without dementia at baseline, found an RR for AD of 1.4, which was not statistically significant after adjustment for other variables, but DM was significantly related to higher risk of a composite outcome of AD and CIND.[7] The risk of AD was also increased in those treated with insulin, indicating a higher risk of AD in subjects with long-standing DM. This study also found a strong association between DM and VD (RR = 3.4). A recent reanalysis of these data, with longer follow-up, showed that the risk of AD associated with DM was stronger than previously reported (RR = 4), independent of other vascular conditions (hypertension, heart disease, stroke) and not explained by misclassification of VD cases as AD.[28]

Few studies have examined if DM in middle age leads to the development of dementia in older age. One study in the USA[29] and another in Israel[30] found that DM at midlife increased the risk of dementia in the elderly. However, a study in Sweden found that DM increased the risk of VD but not of AD,[27] and that this risk was higher in the presence of hypertension and heart disease. Similarly, a study in Japanese-Americans found no association between DM in middle age and AD.[31]

Diabetes mellitus and risk of cognitive decline, MCI and CIND

A small study (20 subjects) showed that acute hyperglycemia is related to worse performance in tests of attention, working memory, and information processing.[32] DM was related to worse decline in 4 years in a verbal fluency test (a test of executive abilities) among 999 participants in the Rancho Bernardo study, but was not related to decline in the MMSE or trail-making tests.[33] A study of 10963 middle-aged and elderly persons showed that DM was a strong predictor of cognitive decline during the 6 years of the study.[34] Another study found similar results.[35] One study showed that DM was associated with worse performance in tests of executive abilities, but not memory.[36] One study among 258 elderly persons without dementia showed that DM was related to a steeper cognitive decline compared with persons without DM, but the decline was more pronounced in persons with both DM and hypertension.[37]

DM has been related to a two-fold higher risk of developing MCI among postmenopausal women.[38] A multiethnic study in the elderly from New York City found that DM was related to a higher risk of CIND with stroke (RR = 2.3), although the effect on CIND without stroke (RR = 1.5) was not evident after adjusting for demographic variables and the presence of the *Apo E-ε4* allele.[7] An Italian study showed a non-statistically significant increase of MCI with DM (RR = 1.4) in an elderly population,[39] while a Canadian study found that DM was related only to vascular CIND.[40]

Diabetes mellitus treatment and cognition

One of the interesting aspects of changes in glucose is that acutely high insulin levels may improve cognition while maintaining euglycemia, while they may worsen it in the long term.[18] In addition, one of the complications of DM treatment is hypoglycemia, which can result in short- and long-term cognitive impairment.[41]

One study of 38 cases of DM and 38 controls found no differences in cognitive performance with DM control, but longer duration of DM was associated with worse performance.[42] Another study of 69 persons with DM and 27 subjects without DM showed that those with DM had worse performance in the MMSE and the digit symbol tests and that, among diabetics, those treated with insulin did worse.[43] Another small study in 19 persons with DM showed that tests of memory were worse among those with poor diabetes control and that ingestion of foods with a high glycemic index further worsened memory at 30 minutes.[44] One study showed that tests of executive function were improved after inpatient treatment in 20 persons with DM.[45] In contrast, a 3-month study in 26 persons with DM failed to show a change in cognition, with improved control mostly achieved with insulin therapy.[46]

A report from 2374 elderly participants in the Nurses Health Study found that women with DM had worse global cognitive performance, and this worsened with longer DM duration.[47] The Nurses Health Study also showed that women with DM treated with oral hypoglycemic agents had cognitive performance similar to those without DM, whereas those diabetics not treated had worse cognitive performance,[48] suggesting that diabetes treatment may improve cognitive performance.

Given that the cognitive problems related to diabetes can be caused by hyperinsulinemia and/or uncontrolled glycemia, it is possible that both glucose control and how it is achieved are important in terms of cognition. It is possible that achieving glucose control through medications that increase insulin levels could be detrimental for cognition in comparison to medications that increase insulin sensitivity thereby decreasing insulin levels. In a randomized study of 145 elderly persons with DM, receiving metformin (an insulin-sensitizing medication), patients that receive either glyburide (a medication that increases insulin levels) or rosiglitazone (a medication that decreases insulin resistance),[49] showed similar improvement in working memory, a frontal task, with better glycemic control.

Impact of cognitive decline in patients with diabetes mellitus

The evidence reviewed above supports that DM is associated with both memory problems and executive problems. The memory problems translate in forgetting appointments, forgetting medications, or taking them more than once if it is forgotten that they were taken. Executive problems include inattention, lack of motivation, and inability to plan and execute a complicated treatment plan. Therefore, these memory and executive impairments may affect proper DM self-care.[50] Fortunately, elderly patients with cognitive impairment receiving a treatment teaching program have shown improved ability in DM self-management,[43] underscoring the need to tailor a treatment plan for persons with DM and cognitive impairment.

Conclusions

Numerous studies have shown an increased risk of dementia and/or cognitive impairment in patients with DM. This relationship seems to be stronger for the vascular cognitive syndromes, but also exists for AD. In addition to the strong epidemiologic data, laboratory data show that the association between DM and cognitive impairment is biologically plausible. The cognitive profile of persons with DM can be expected to include short-term memory impairment, problems with memory retrieval, inattention, low motivation, and with organizational abilities. The fact that DM increases cognitive impairment raises concerns about the ability of persons with this disorder to follow proper treatment. There are data suggesting that better DM control improves cognition, but more studies are necessary to address this issue.

Acknowledgements

Dr Luchsinger's work is supported by grants from the National Institutes of Health AG07232, AG07702, 1K08AG20856-01, and from the Alzheimer's Association IIRG-05-15053.

Dr Florez's work is supported by grants from the Department of Veterans Affairs Miami GRECC and CSP#465, Pan American Health Organization RC/RG-T/VEN/3201, and UM-Humana Health Service Research, and National Institutes of Health NIDDK DK01 0500.

References

1. Luchsinger J, Mayeux R. Cardiovascular risk factors and Alzheimer's disease. Curr Atheroscler Rep 2004; 6: 261–6.
2. Harris MI. Diabetes in America: epidemiology and scope of the problem. Diabetes Care 1998; 21(Suppl 3): C11–14.
3. Luchsinger JA. Diabetes. In: Aguirre-Molina M, Molina CW, Zambrana RE, eds. Health Issues in the Latino Community, CA. San Francisco, CA. Jossey Bass, 2001: 277–300.
4. Ritchie K, Lovestone S. The dementias. Lancet 2002; 360(9347): 1759–66.
5. Petersen RC. Mild cognitive impairment as a diagnostic entity. J Intern Med 2004; 256(3): 183–94.
6. Luis CA, Loewenstein DA, Acevedo A, Barker WW, Duara R. Mild cognitive impairment: directions for future research. Neurology 2003; 61: 438–44.
7. Luchsinger JA, Tang MX, Stern Y, Shea S, Mayeux R. Diabetes mellitus and risk of Alzheimer's disease and dementia with stroke in a multiethnic cohort. Am J Epidemiol 2001; 154: 635–41.
8. Folstein MF, Folstein SE, McHugh PR. 'Mini-mental state'. A practical method for grading the cognitive state of patients for the clinician. J Psychiatr Res 1975; 12: 189–98.
9. Small SA, Mayeux R. A clinical approach to memory decline. J Pract Psychiatry Behav Health 1999; 5: 87–94.
10. Royall DR, Lauterbach EC, Cummings JL et al. Executive control function: a review of its promise and challenges for clinical research. A report from the Committee on Research of the American Neuropsychiatric Association. J Neuropsychiatry Clin Neurosci 2002; 14: 377–405.
11. Royall D. The 'Alzheimerization' of dementia research. J Am Geriatr Soc 2003; 51(2): 277–78.

12. Karapanayiotides T, Piechowski-Jozwiak B, van Melle G, Bogousslavsky J, Devuyst G. Stroke patterns, etiology, and prognosis in patients with diabetes mellitus. Neurology 2004; 62(9): 1558–62.
13. Serra JA, Marschoff ER, Dominguez RO et al. Collaborative Group for the Study of the Oxidative Stress, Argentina. Oxidative stress in Alzheimer's and vascular dementias: masking of the antioxidant profiles by a concomitant Type II diabetes mellitus condition. J Neurol Sci 2004; 218: 17–24.
14. Yamagishi S, Nakamura K, Inoue H, Kikuchi S, Takeuchi M. Serum or cerebrospinal fluid levels of glyceraldehyde-derived advanced glycation end products (AGEs) may be a promising biomarker for early detection of Alzheimer's disease. Med Hypotheses 2005; 64: 1205–7.
15. Strachan MWJ. Insulin and cognitive function. Lancet 2003; 362: 1253.
16. Farris W, Mansourian S, Chang Y et al. Insulin-degrading enzyme regulates the levels of insulin, amyloid beta-protein, and the beta-amyloid precursor protein intracellular domain in vivo. Proc Natl Acad Sci USA 2003; 100: 4162–7.
17. Watson GS, Bernhardt T, Reger MA et al. Insulin effects on CSF norepinephrine and cognition in Alzheimer's disease. Neurobiol Aging 2006; 27: 38–41.
18. Watson GS, Craft S. Modulation of memory by insulin and glucose: neuropsychological observations in Alzheimer's disease. Eur J Pharmacol 2004; 490: 97–113.
19. Janson J, Laedtke T, Parisi JE et al. Increased risk of type 2 diabetes in Alzheimer disease. Diabetes 2004; 53: 474–81.
20. Beeri MS, Silverman JM, Davis KL et al. Type 2 diabetes is negatively associated with Alzheimer's disease neuropathology. J Gerontol A Biol Sci Med Sci 2005; 60: 471–75.
21. Yoshitake T, Kiyohara Y, Kato I et al. Incidence and risk factors of vascular dementia and Alzheimer's disease in a defined elderly Japanese population: the Hisayama Study. Neurology 1995; 45: 1161–8.
22. Ott A, Stolk RP, van Harskamp F et al. Diabetes mellitus and the risk of dementia: The Rotterdam Study. Neurology 1999; 53: 1937–42.
23. Brayne C, Gill C, Huppert FA et al. Vascular risks and incident dementia: results from a cohort study of the very old. Dement Geriatr Cogn Disord 1998; 9: 175–80.
24. Leibson CL, Rocca WA, Hanson VA et al. Risk of dementia among persons with diabetes mellitus: a population-based cohort study. Am J Epidemiol 1997; 145: 301–8.
25. Arvanitakis Z, Wilson RS, Bienias JL, Evans DA, Bennett DA. Diabetes mellitus and risk of Alzheimer disease and decline in cognitive function. Arch Neurol 2004; 61: 661–6.
26. Peila R, Rodriguez BL, Launer LJ, Honolulu–Asia Aging Study. Type 2 diabetes, APOE gene, and the risk for dementia and related pathologies: The Honolulu–Asia Aging Study. Diabetes 2002; 51: 1256–62.
27. Xu WL, Qiu CX, Wahlin A, Winblad B, Fratiglioni L. Diabetes mellitus and risk of dementia in the Kungsholmen project: a 6-year follow-up study. Neurology 2004; 63: 1181–6.
28. Luchsinger JA, Reitz C, Honig LS et al. Aggregation of vascular risk factors and risk of incident Alzheimer disease. Neurology 2005; 65: 545–51.
29. Whitmer RA, Sidney S, Selby J, Johnston SC, Yaffe K. Midlife cardiovascular risk factors and risk of dementia in late life. Neurology 2005; 64: 277–81.
30. Schnaider Beeri M, Goldbourt U, Silverman JM et al. Diabetes mellitus in midlife and the risk of dementia three decades later. Neurology 2004; 63: 1902–7.
31. Curb JD, Rodriguez BL, Abbott RD et al. Longitudinal association of vascular and Alzheimer's dementias, diabetes, and glucose tolerance. Neurology 1999; 52: 971–5.

32. Sommerfield AJ, Deary IJ, Frier BM. Acute hyperglycemia alters mood state and impairs cognitive performance in people with type 2 diabetes. Diabetes Care 2004; 27: 2335–40.

33. Kanaya AM, Barrett-Connor E, Gildengorin G, Yaffe K. Change in cognitive function by glucose tolerance status in older adults: a 4-year prospective study of the Rancho Bernardo study cohort. Arch Intern Med 2004; 164: 1327–33.

34. Knopman D, Boland LL, Mosley T et al. Cardiovascular risk factors and cognitive decline in middle-aged adults. Neurology 2001; 56: 42–8.

35. Fontbonne A, Berr C, Ducimetiere P, Alperovitch A. Changes in cognitive abilities over a 4-year period are unfavorably affected in elderly diabetic subjects: results of the Epidemiology of Vascular Aging Study. Diabetes Care 2001; 24: 366–70.

36. Vanhanen M, Kuusisto J, Koivisto K et al. Type-2 diabetes and cognitive function in a non-demented population. Acta Neurol Scand 1999; 100: 97–101.

37. Hassing LB, Hofer SM, Nilsson SE et al. Comorbid type 2 diabetes mellitus and hypertension exacerbates cognitive decline: evidence from a longitudinal study. Age Ageing 2004; 33: 355–61.

38. Yaffe K, Blackwell T, Kanaya AM et al. Diabetes, impaired fasting glucose, and development of cognitive impairment in older women. Neurology 2004; 63: 658–63.

39. Solfrizzi V, Panza F, Colacicco AM et al. Vascular risk factors, incidence of MCI, and rates of progression to dementia. Neurology 2004; 63: 1882–91.

40. MacKnight C, Rockwood K, Awalt E, McDowell I. Diabetes mellitus and the risk of dementia, Alzheimer's disease and vascular cognitive impairment in the Canadian Study of Health and Aging. Dement Geriatr Cogn Disord 2002; 14: 77–83.

41. Strachan MW, Deary IJ, Ewing FM, Frier BM. Recovery of cognitive function and mood after severe hypoglycemia in adults with insulin-treated diabetes. Diabetes Care 2000; 23: 305–12.

42. Cosway R, Strachan MW, Dougall A, Frier BM, Deary IJ. Cognitive function and information processing in type 2 diabetes. Diabet Med 2001; 18: 803–10.

43. Mogi N, Umegaki H, Hattori A et al. Cognitive function in Japanese elderly with type 2 diabetes mellitus. J Diabetes Complications 2004; 18: 42–6.

44. Greenwood CE, Kaplan RJ, Hebblethwaite S, Jenkins DJ. Carbohydrate-induced memory impairment in adults with type 2 diabetes. Diabetes Care 2003; 26: 1961–6.

45. Naor M, Steingruber HJ, Westhoff K, Schottenfeld-Naor Y, Gries AF. Cognitive function in elderly non-insulin-dependent diabetic patients before and after inpatient treatment for metabolic control. J Diabetes Complications 1997; 11: 40–6.

46. Mussell M, Hewer W, Kulzer B, Bergis K, Rist F. Effects of improved glycaemic control maintained for 3 months on cognitive function in patients with Type 2 diabetes. Diabet Med 2004; 21: 1253–6.

47. Grodstein F, Chen J, Wilson RS, Manson JE. Type 2 diabetes and cognitive function in community-dwelling elderly women. Diabetes Care 2001; 24: 1060–5.

48. Logroscino G, Kang JH, Grodstein F. Prospective study of type 2 diabetes and cognitive decline in women aged 70–81 years. BMJ 2004; 328(7439): 548.

49. Ryan CM, Freed MI, Rood JA et al. Improving metabolic control leads to better working memory in adults with type 2 diabetes. Diabetes Care 2006; 29: 345–51.

50. Sinclair AJ, Girling AJ, Bayer AJ. Cognitive dysfunction in older subjects with diabetes mellitus: impact on diabetes self-management and use of care services. All Wales Research into Elderly (AWARE) Study. Diabetes Res Clin Pract 2000; 50: 203–12.

Chapter 5

Diabetes mellitus and sexual dysfunction

Marilyn Sanjuan-Horvath

Introduction

Both physiological and psychological factors can contribute to sexual dysfunction among patients with diabetes mellitus (DM). Often, patients may be unaware that sexual dysfunction is a symptom of a co-occurring psychiatric disorder, a consequence of medical illness, or a side effect of psychotropic medications. Additionally, patients may feel uncomfortable voicing their concerns with their provider. Clinicians need to initiate the discussion to facilitate early identification of problems and offer treatment options. This chapter will review the types of sexual dysfunction commonly associated with DM and currently available approaches to their evaluation and treatment.

Normal sexual response

In order to recognize and assess sexual dysfunction, a basic understanding of normal sexual response is helpful. Normal human sexual activity is often described as composed of four physiological and psychological stages: desire, arousal, orgasm, and resolution. *Desire,* or libido, is a psychological urge, modulated by several neurotransmitters, including serotonin, dopamine, norepinephrine, and prolactin. Additionally, normal testosterone levels, in both men and women, are associated with enhanced desire. During the *arousal* phase, muscle tone increases, and several physical responses occur, including penile erection in men, vasocongestion and lubrication of the vaginal area, and swelling of the clitoris and breasts in women. In men, *orgasm* consists of contractions of the prostate, seminal vesicles, and urethra,

Table 5.1   Changes in phases of sexual functioning associated with aging

Stage	Men	Women
Desire	• Declines with decreasing testosterone levels	• Declines with menopausal, symptoms and with declining testosterone levels
Arousal	• Requires greater tactile stimulation • Erections take longer to achieve and not as rigid	• Decreased vaginal blood flow with less swelling • Less vaginal lubrication • Decreased clitoral and breast sensitivity • Requires greater tactile stimulation
Orgasm	• Takes longer to achieve • Requires more stimulation • Contractions are less intense • Decreased volume of ejaculate	• Takes longer to achieve • Requires more stimulation • Contractions are less intense
Resolution	• Prolonged	• Prolonged

and leads to ejaculation. Contractions of the muscles of the outer third of the vagina occur in women. Generalized muscular tension, perineal contractions, and rhythmic involuntary pelvic thrusting also typically occur in both sexes. It is experienced as a sensation of euphoria. During *resolution*, both men and women experience a psychological sense of relaxation and well-being, and men are refractory to further orgasm for variable durations. Women, on the other hand, may continue to be responsive to additional stimulation.

There are many factors, including age (Table 5.1), that can interfere with one or several of these stages, leading to sexual symptoms. The types of problems that are reported vary by gender. Psychiatric disorders and psychosocial stressors can interfere with normal sexual responses, and lead to sexual dysfunction. Loss of libido itself is a frequent symptom of depressive and anxiety disorders, and can result from alcohol and other CNS depressant abuse. Similarly, the microvascular changes that result from DM are associated with difficulties in several stages of sexual response. For example, erectile dysfunction is often a presenting symptom of previously undetected diabetes. Lastly, many medications used to treat medical and psychiatric disorders can lead to decreased libido, lowered sexual response, erectile dysfunction, retrograde ejaculation, and anorgasmia (Table 5.2).

Sexual dysfunction in men

Sexual dysfunction typically increases with age, with 20–30% of adult men reporting some type of sexual dysfunction. By far, the most commonly reported sexual problem in men is erectile dysfunction (ED). ED is defined as the inability to achieve or sustain an erection that is adequate for sexual function. Worldwide, in 1995, there were over 152 million men who experienced ED.[1] By 2025, worldwide prevalence of ED is expected to number 322 million, an increase of nearly 170 million men.[1] The risk of ED increases with age, lower education, diabetes, heart disease, hypertension,[2] and tobacco use.[3]

Causes of erectile dysfunction

Following arousal, the brain activates the parasympathetic system to relax the penile smooth muscle tissue through release of nitric oxide and activation of cyclic guanosine monophosphate (cGMP). As the muscles relax, blood flow increases, expanding the corpora cavernosa (the two cylindrical sponge-like structures that run the length of the penis), which straightens and stiffens the penis. With ejaculation, the enzyme phosphodiesterase type 5 (PDE5) breaks down cGMP, leading to smooth muscle contraction. The excess blood drains out of the corpora, and the penis returns to its flaccid state. At least 80% of ED is due to a problem that affects one of these factors: failure of arousal, impaired neurologic response, or impaired vascular response.[4]

A variety of risk factors can contribute or worsen ED (Table 5.3). Chronic medical illness can cause loss of interest in sex, fatigue, and can keep adequate blood flow from reaching the penis. Bladder, rectal, or prostate cancer surgeries and spinal cord injuries can damage parasympathetic nerves and cause ED. Prolonged bicycle riding can also temporarily cause ED. Medications, due to a variety of mechanisms (see Table 5.2), can contribute to ED through either impairment of the neurologic or vascular processes. Chronic alcohol use, and concomitant nutritional deficiencies, can interfere with neurologic functioning. Chronic tobacco use can damage penile arteries.

Table 5.2   Medications associated with sexual dysfunction and alternatives in patients with diabetes

Drug class	Medications associated with sexual dysfunction	Alternatives with less sexual dysfunction
Antihypertensives:		
• β-blocker	• Atenolol, labetalol, metoprolol, propranolol	ACE inhibitors:
• α₁-antagonist	• Prazosin, doxazosin	• Captopril, enalapril, lisinopril, benazepril, quinapril
• α₂-agonist	• Clonidine	
• Diuretics	• HCTZ, amiloride, spironolactone	
Antipsychotics:		
• Conventionals	• Chlorpromazine, haloperidol, perphenazine, thioridazine	Atypicals:
• Atypical	• Risperidone	• Aripiprazole, quetiapine, ziprasidone
Antidepressants:		
• SSRIs	• Fluoxetine, sertraline, paroxetine, citalopram	• Bupropion, mirtazapine
• TCAs	• Imipramine, desipramine, nortriptyline	
Anticonvulsants	• Carbamazepine, phenytoin, valproic acid	• Oxcarbazepine, lamotrigine

HCTZ, hydrochlorothiazide; ACE inhibitors, angiotensin-converting enzyme inhibitors; SSRIs: selective serotonin reuptake inhibitors; TCAs, tricyclic antidepressants.

Table 5.3   Risk factors associated with erectile dysfunction and physiologic component affected

Risk factor	Arousal	Neurologic response	Vascular response
Chronic medical illness:			
• Diabetes		×	×
• Atherosclerosis	×	×	×
• COPD	×		×
• Hormonal changes	×		
Surgery or trauma	×	×	
Medications		×	×
Alcohol, marijuana	×		×
Tobacco			×
Stress, anxiety, depression	×		×

COPD, chronic obstructive pulmonary disease.

A few cases of ED may still be associated with psychological causes. These primarily include stress, anxiety, and fatigue. Additionally, having negative feelings toward the sexual partner such as anger, loss of interest, and resentment can lead to ED. Similarly, negative feelings expressed by the sexual partner, such as criticism and hostility, may be contributory factors. Physical and psychological factors often interact. For example, as a man ages, the sexual response slows, and this may cause self-doubt about the ability to attain an erection. The anxiety can then increase, leading to greater difficulty in obtaining the erection.

Sexual dysfunction, depression, and diabetes mellitus

Men with depression had an almost two-fold increased likelihood of having moderate or complete ED compared with non-depressed men.[5] Similarly, sexual dysfunction is prevalent among men with diabetes, occurring two to four times more often than in persons without diabetes.[4,6,7] Whereas ED most commonly develops after the age of 60 years, it tends to occur 5–10 years earlier among men with diabetes,[8] with a slightly lower prevalence among men with type 1 DM (32% vs 46% in men with type 2 DM).[9]

There are several interesting hypotheses to explain the relationship between ED, depression, and DM. One possibility is that one disease causes the other two. Nocturnal penile tumescence (NPT) is lost during depressive episodes, suggesting that depression may somehow interfere with normal erectile function.[10] Decreased libido, ED, and decreased sexual activity are all well-recognized symptoms of depressive illness. Depression and diabetes are known to co-occur with increased frequency, so that men with diabetes are more likely to be depressed than non-diabetics, and therefore, ED is more likely to occur. Alternatively, depression may be a psychologically reactive consequence of having ED, and since diabetes is a risk factor for ED[8] there would be a higher co-occurrence of the three disorders.[11] In this case, successful treatment of ED should lead to decreased depressive symptoms, and several randomized trials have now shown this to be the case.[12–14]

A second theory suggests that depression, DM, and ED share common pathophysiologies, and the most likely etiologies are age and vascular disease. DM, ED, and certain depressive syndromes occur more commonly with age. After the age of 60 years, most men with DM are affected by ED.[15] DM and depression are both recognized risk factors for vascular disease,[16] which is the most common cause of ED.[17] Longer duration of DM is associated with more vascular complications, including ED. Duration of DM > 10 years is associated with a three times greater likelihood of ED compared with duration < 5 years.[18] Vascular disease has also been implicated as causative in a type of depression known as vascular depression, which typically presents after the age of 60. Lastly, depression is associated with poorer DM outcomes, and higher levels of hemoglobin A_{1c} (HbA$_{1c}$). There is a clear association between poor glucose control, high HbA$_{1c}$ levels, and the presence of ED.[19] Men with diabetic complications were more likely to report sexual dysfunction than those without such complications.

Sexual dysfunction, schizophrenia, and diabetes mellitus

Patients with schizophrenia are at increased risk for DM compared with the general population. They also typically have poorer medical outcomes than the general population, so that it would be likely that men with schizophrenia and DM would exhibit a higher prevalence of sexual dysfunction. There is a surprising paucity of literature on this topic. Among men with untreated schizophrenia, the most commonly reported sexual problem is decreased desire, but some studies have suggested that sexual dysfunction occurs in as many as 54% of men with schizophrenia.[20–22] Those patients who report dysfunction also had lower ratings on quality of life measures, and were less likely to have a romantic partner. Among men with schizophrenia who had a partner, the quality of the relationship was described as poor. Sexual dysfunction in this population is associated with elevated prolactin levels, usually as a side effect of antipsychotic medications. Some of these medications are also associated with increasing the risk for DM and dyslipidemias, so that it is unclear if the sexual dysfunction is related to either schizophrenia or DM, or both conditions.

Sexual dysfunction in women

Sexual concerns can occur at any age in women, but primarily take place during times of hormonal changes, such as pregnancy, postpartum, and menopause, and in conjunction with various illnesses, such as cardiovascular disease and diabetes. More than 40% of women will report sexual dysfunction.[23,24] The sexual disorders reported include *sexual desire disorders, sexual arousal disorders, orgasmic disorders,* and *sexual pain disorders.*[25] *Hypoactive sexual desire disorder,* the most frequently reported disorder, is defined as persistently deficient sexual fantasies and desire for sexual activity. *Sexual arousal disorder* is the inability to attain or maintain an adequate lubrication-swelling response of sexual excitement until completion of sexual activity. *Orgasmic disorder* is a delay in, or absence of, orgasm following the normal sexual excitement phase. This diagnosis is based on the clinician's judgment that the patient's orgasmic capacity is less than would be reasonable given her age, sexual experience, and adequacy of stimulation. Sexual pain disorders are typically of two types, dyspareunia and vaginismus. Dyspareunia is genital pain associated with sexual intercourse which is not exclusively caused by lack of lubrication. Dyspareunia may be superficial, vaginal, or deep. Superficial dyspareunia occurs with attempted penetration and is usually related to anatomic or irritative conditions. Vaginal dyspareunia is pain related to friction from insufficient lubrication. Deep dyspareunia is related to thrusting, and is often associated with pelvic disease or relaxation. Vaginismus is an involuntary spasm of the musculature of the outer third of the vagina which interferes with sexual intercourse. In order for any of these symptom clusters to meet criteria for a disorder, the symptoms must cause marked distress or interpersonal difficulty, and are not due to another psychiatric disorder or general medical condition or the physiological effects of a medication or substance of abuse.

Causes of sexual dysfunction

As seen in men, anything that interferes with desire and arousal, or impairs the neurologic or vascular responses that are necessary for normal sexual functioning in women, can lead to sexual dysfunction. A variety of physiologic changes associated with sexual functioning occur as women age (see Table 5.1). Although many of these changes are attributed to estrogen deficiency, decreased testosterone serum levels can also lead to fatigue, loss of libido, and decreased genital and nipple sensitivity. Additionally, several medical conditions and/or their treatments, including diabetes, hypertension, depression, cancer, pelvic surgery, and multiple sclerosis, can lead to a decreased libido or difficulty achieving orgasm. Dyspareunia commonly occurs after menopause because genital tissue becomes atrophied, with reduced labial swelling and lubrication.

Table 5.4 describes the major psychological variables that contribute to female sexual dysfunction. The experience a woman has had with sexual partners can affect her desire for and ability to respond appropriately in a sexual situation. Women with a history of prior physical or sexual abuse often exhibit sexual disorders. Sexual dysfunction is a frequent symptom of depressive and anxiety disorders,[24] or may occur as a side effect of some antidepressant medications. Marital discord often co-occurs with symptoms of anxiety, depression, and sexual dysfunction.[24] At times, women may find competing roles difficult to balance, such as work demands, and caring for children or an aging parent, which can lead to stress, feelings of anger or resentment, and fatigue, all of which can interfere with sexual responsiveness. Lastly, the health and age of the sexual partner can lead to sexual dissatisfaction. Frequently, the cause of female sexual dysfunction is multifactorial and interconnected.

Sexual dysfunction and diabetes mellitus

Sexual dysfunction in women with diabetes has been much less studied than in men. Women with diabetes are twice as likely as non-diabetic

Table 5.4   Psychological variables that can contribute to female
sexual dysfunction

Psychological variable	Factors
Sexual or emotional abuse	• Child abuse • Domestic violence • Sexual exploitation • Trust issues • Desensitization
Depression	• Symptom of major depressive disorder • Grief • Secondary to antidepressants
Relationship issues	• Negative sexual experiences • Religious, cultural, or social conflicts with partner • Different sexual preferences • Marital conflicts
Stress	• Job vs homemaking vs caregiver duties • Financial problems • Infertility
Self-esteem	• Weight gain • Aging • Poor self-image • Insulin injections

women to experience sexual dysfunction.[26] In general, women with type 1 DM report fewer sexual problems (27%) than do those with type 2 DM (42%),[27,28] but both groups of diabetic women report more dysfunction than controls. Also, because type 1 DM begins at an earlier age, this difference may be due to the younger age of study participants of the type 1 groups. Among those with type 1 DM, sexual dysfunction has been related to depression and the quality of the partner relationship.[29]

Women with type 2 DM report decreased sexual desire, decreased frequency of orgasm, reduced vaginal lubrication, and dyspareunia.[30] The most commonly reported problem, an issue highlighted in most studies, was reduced vaginal lubrication. Unlike men, duration of diabetes does not appear to affect sexual functioning in women. Women with diabetic complications report more sexual dysfunction problems (33%) than women without complications (22%). Diabetes may affect arousal due to decreased genital sensation and lubrication. Women with type 2 DM are also predisposed to vaginal dryness and infections, which can lead to dyspareunia. Again, the overall poorer quality of the marital relationship and more depressive symptoms in diabetic women are associated with sexual dysfunction.[31]

Evaluation of sexual dysfunction

Interview

The evaluation of sexual dysfunction relies on the clinician being knowledgeable and comfortable inquiring about sexual functioning and problems. The clinician must be able to ask direct questions, using language the patient can understand. At times, the clinician may also have to provide education, including terms for the phases of normal sexual activity, to some patients. An interview with the sexual partner, in the presence of the affected person, may also be very helpful. An effective method of facilitating open lines of communication regarding sexual issues is to use a formal interview. The goal is to identify problems that may be occurring, recognize the phases of the sexual response that are affected, and determine likely causes for those problems.

Several scales have been developed which can be incorporated into a routine initial visit.[32–34] In working with a diabetic man, questions regarding erectile function are particularly pertinent, including: can you get an erection; do you have morning erections; are you able to have erections while masturbating but not during sex; are you able to have erections with one partner, but not another. For diabetic women, inquiry should include questions about any problems with desire, arousal, lubrication, pain during intercourse, or orgasms, and the quality of their marital relationship. Equally important is to have an understanding of the person's sexual history, including questions about the person's beliefs and fears regarding sexuality, any sexual problems they had in the past, and safe sex practices.

Both men and women with diabetes should be screened for depressive and other psychiatric symptoms (psychosis, anxiety, substance use disorders) that may be interfering with desire or arousal. Women, in particular, should be screened for a history of sexual or physical trauma. Additionally, a surgical history (prostatic, gynecologic, pelvic) is important, as is a medical history, in that at times, sexual dysfunction is the presenting symptom of a medical condition, including diabetes. Lastly, a review of the patient's medications is important, since several drug classes are associated with sexual disorders (see Table 5.2).

Physical and laboratory evaluations

A complete physical examination, with particular attention to the urologic and gynecologic systems, is needed. This may identify a vaginal infection or a sexually transmitted disease as the cause of the dysfunction. Laboratory tests include:

- fasting glucose (to identify new cases of diabetes)
- lipid profile (risk factor for vascular disease)
- thyroid functions
- testosterone and prolactin serum levels
- prostate-specific antigen (PSA) in men
- follicle-stimulating hormone (FSH) and luteinizing hormone (LH) in women.

Treatment of sexual dysfunction

The primary goal of treatment is to determine the etiology of the sexual dysfunction and treat it whenever possible. If the primary problem is a newly diagnosed medical condition, such as diabetes or hypothyroidism, treating the underlying condition may improve the sexual problem. If the sexual dysfunction is a symptom of a depressive, anxiety, or psychotic disorder, the patient should be referred for treatment of the underlying psychiatric disorder.

Education

Education regarding sexual health should be an important part of diabetes disease self-management. For example, Mellinger notes that high school seniors with diabetes should be prepared for life at college and know that sexual activity can lower blood glucose levels.[35] Also, a discussion should occur to address concerns about ED, either because some young men may be experiencing it or are worried about the possibility of it in the future. Similarly, self-esteem and self-image should be discussed with diabetic women. If obesity is present, appropriate nutritional and exercise instruction should be provided. Safe-sex practices also need to be discussed with all patients. Patients with diabetes may have co-occurring psychiatric illness, which is associated with an increased risk for human immunodeficiency virus (HIV) infection. Many of the treatments for HIV are associated with inducing metabolic disturbances, and may worsen glycemic control. Additionally, diabetic patients may be more susceptible to some sexually transmitted diseases, as their immune systems may be compromised.

Psychotherapy

The main goals of psychotherapy for sexual dysfunction are to correct sexual misinformation, enhance partner communication and honesty, reduce anxiety, improve sensual experience and pleasure, and facilitate interpersonal tolerance and acceptance. Partners are encouraged to discuss their sexual preferences, changes that they are experiencing, and problems. They are supported to deal with anger and resentment directly. Recommendations are made to the partners to spend relaxed time together with and without sexual activity. Examples of this type of activity can include warm baths, relaxation, yoga, meditation, and massage. Individual psychotherapy may be indicated when a psychiatric disorder is identified or to address unresolved conflicts.

Managing medication-related sexual dysfunction

The first step is to determine that the sexual dysfunction is truly related to the medication, and not due to another cause. If the medication was recently started, tolerance to the side effect may develop, so simply waiting 1–2 weeks may resolve the problem. A change to an alternate medication that is less associated with sexual side effects may be needed (see Table 5.2). For example, the conventional neuroleptics and risperidone cause sexual symptoms by raising prolactin levels. Preferred antipsychotics in diabetic patients include aripiprazole, ziprasidone, and quetiapine. For α_1-antagonists, α_2-agonists, and β-blockers, angiotensin-converting enzyme (ACE) inhibitors may be preferred antihypertensive agents. For antidepressants, bupropion and mirtazapine are preferred drugs. If there is a clinical reason that the antidepressant cannot be switched, sildenafil effectively improves erectile function and other aspects of sexual function in men with sexual dysfunction associated with the use of selective serotonin reuptake inhibitors (SSRIs).[36,37]

Treatment options for male sexual dysfunction

If ED is primary, there are five generally accepted and approved types of treatments: oral medications, the vacuum constriction devices, intracavernosal injection therapy, intraurethral therapy, and penile prostheses. All treatment options are effective, but a satisfactory treatment for one patient may be unsatisfactory for another. The advantages and disadvantages for each will be weighed differently, based on individual patient preference as well as the preference of the sexual partner.

Oral medications

Phosphodiesterase type 5 inhibitors

In 1985, scientists at Pfizer Inc. developed a medication to treat heart failure and hypertension. Several years later, healthy study subjects reported more frequent erections after taking the medication. In March of 1998 the US Food and Drug Administration (FDA) approved the use of Viagra (sildenafil citrate) to treat ED. The enzyme PDE5 hydrolyzes the breakdown of cGMP in the corpora cavernosa. Inhibition of PDE5 results in vasodilation, increased arterial blood flow, smooth muscle relaxation, and penile erection. Three PDE5 inhibitors are currently approved by the US. FDA for the treatment of ED: sildenafil, vardenafil, and tadalafil. These are currently first-line treatment choices for most cases of primary ED.

Sildenafil (Viagra) was the first PDE5 inhibitor approved, with more than 23 million men treated over a 7-year post marketing time frame.[38] Effective dosages are 25, 50, and 100 mg. The starting dose should be 50 mg, adjusted according to the response and side effects. It becomes effective after 30–60 minutes, has a duration of action of about 5 hours, and its effect may be reduced by heavy fatty meals. It has been specifically studied in both types 1 and 2 DM men and found to be well-tolerated and improved erections in 56–66% of the men studied.[39,40]

Vardenafil (Levitra) in vitro is more potent than sildenafil, but this does not necessarily imply greater clinical efficacy. It is available in 5, 10, and 20 mg doses. The starting dose should be 10 mg, adjusted according to the response and side effects. It is effective after 30 minutes, with a duration of action of about 5 hours. Its effect may be reduced by heavy fatty meals. Vardenafil has been found to significantly improve erectile function in men with types 1 and 2 DM, and was generally well-tolerated.[41] The 20 mg dose was effective for 72% of study participants, compared with 57% of responders in the 10 mg group.

Tadalafil (Cialis) is available in 10 and 20 mg doses. The starting dose should be 10 mg, adjusted according to the response and side effects. It is effective after 30 minutes, with a duration of action from 24 to 36 hours. Unlike the other PDE5 inhibitors, it is not influenced by food or alcohol. It has been found to significantly enhance erectile function in men with both types 1 and 2 DM, and was well-tolerated.[42,43] PDE5 inhibitors share the following common side effects: headaches, dizziness, flushing, dyspepsia, nasal congestion, rhinitis, visual disturbance, back pain, and myalgias. Men with diabetes are consistently found to have more severe ED than non-diabetic men. In all studies of PDE5 inhibitors, while men with diabetes do respond to these medications, their response is slightly lower than in men without diabetes. Studies have yet to investigate the use of one drug in the event of treatment failure with one of the other agents.

The PDE5 inhibitors are contraindicated in patients taking nitrates, and relatively contraindicated in patients with active coronary ischemia, recent heart attack, stroke, arrhythmias, congestive heart failure, border-line low blood pressure, low cardiac volume status, and/or a complicated multidrug antihypertensive therapies. Inhibitors of CYP3A4, such as erythromycin, ketoconazole, protease inhibitors, and delavirdine, used in the treatment of patients with HIV, can increase the levels of PDE5 inhibitors. If a PDE5 is to be used in this population, the smallest starting dose should be considered. Patients should also be warned not to combine them with oral recreational nitrates, including 'poppers'. The combination can induce severe hypotension, which could be fatal.

Apomorphine sublingual (Uprima, Ixense, Taluvian)

This medication is not approved for the treatment of ED by the FDA in the USA. It has been registered in other countries since 2002 for treatment of ED, however.[44] It is a sublingual dopaminergic agonist that acts to enhance proerectile stimuli through the hypothalamic neural pathways. It produces a rapid circulating plasma concentration, resulting in a quick onset of action, producing an erection in a median time of 18–20 minutes. The main side effect is nausea. There are no reported interactions with other medications, food, and alcohol.[45,46] This medication has been studied in diabetic men with inconclusive results.[47,48]

Vacuum constrictive devices

In 1917, Otto Ledever obtained a patent for a penile vacuum device. The penis was inserted into a tube, then air is extracted leading to negative pressure that caused engorgement of the penis. In 1982, the FDA approved the use of a vacuum constrictive device (VCD) to treat ED. VCDs consist of a plastic cylinder, a vacuum pump, and an elastic constriction band. A lubricant is applied to the penis, and the cylinder is placed over it. Air is pumped out of the cylinder, which creates a vacuum, causing an erection. The constriction band is then transferred to the base of the erect penis to maintain the erection. The cylinder is then removed. The constriction band can be left on the penis safely for about 30 minutes. After intercourse, the band is removed. Approximately three-quarters of men who began using the VCD (prior to availability of medications for ED) continued to use it. Most drop-outs occur in the first 3 months of treatment. The most commonly reported problems are interruption of intercourse, and some men complain of numbness or coldness of the penis and/or discomfort upon ejaculation. Side effects include penile pain, bruising, and trapped ejaculation. Use of anticoagulant therapy is a relative contraindication.

Intracavernosal injection therapy

Vasoactive medications are injected in the corpora cavernosa, which dilates the penile arteries and relaxes penile tissue. Blood flow increases cause an erection. The medications used include alprostadil or prostaglandin E_1 (PGE_1) alone or in combination with other drugs (papaverine, phentolamine). Only two drugs are currently FDA approved: alprostadil sterile powder (Caverject) and alprostadil alfadex (Edex).[44] Often, the first injection occurs at the physician's office to determine how well the penis will respond. Erections occur within 5–15 minutes after the injection, and can last 1 hour or more. Patients usually tolerate the procedure well, with minimal pain complaints. Most treatment drop-outs occur in the first 2 months. The most serious side effect is an erection that is prolonged, lasting more than 4 hours. The risk of a prolonged erection is 1–8%, but may be lower in patients who follow instruction, and have proper dosage adjustments. Rarely, scar tissue may form at the injection site. Patient education and comfort are essential in the practice of intracavernosal injection therapy. There is an automatic pen that avoids the needle view for those patients who experience fear of the penile puncture. Injection therapy is contraindicated in men with a history of hypersensitivity to the drug used, patients with sickle cell anemia, and in men at risk of developing priapism. It is also not advised in men with limited manual dexterity; however, their partners may be taught the technique if they are willing. This therapy is effective in 60–90% of patients.

Self-administered intraurethral therapy

This method is also known as medicated urethral system for erection (MUSE). With this method a disposable applicator is used to insert a tiny suppository about half the size of a grain of rice about 2 inches into the urethra. The suppository is absorbed by the erectile tissue in the penis, causing increased blood flow that leads to an erection. Side effects include pain, minor bleeding in the urethra, and hypotension.[44] It may cause vaginal irritation, and condoms should be used with partners who are pregnant.

Prosthesis or penile implants

This treatment option is often a last resort because it is invasive and irreversible. It is reserved for select cases that fail other treatment modalities. A penile prosthesis is a plastic device, surgically implanted inside the penis. Two types of prostheses exist: a malleable, semi-rigid rod and an inflatable. The inflatable penile prosthesis provides a more cosmetic erection and has higher rates of patient and partner satisfaction. Inflatable prostheses can have one, two, or three pieces. Fluid is pumped from a reservoir into two implanted cylinders, which stiffen the penis. Pressing a valve at the base of the pump returns the fluid to the reservoir, deflating the cylinders. Penile implant surgery is uncommonly associated with prosthesis infection (1–5%), but may result in scarring and penile deformity. Mechanical failures occur in approximately 1 out of 10 inflatable prostheses and in 1 of 20 malleable prostheses.

Treatment options for female sexual dysfunction

A variety of treatment options are available for female sexual dysfunction. Few of these treatments have been specifically studied in diabetic populations. The treatments are targeted towards the specific type of disorder.

Hypoactive sexual desire disorder

There are no FDA-approved medications to treat this disorder. Estrogen replacement therapy may be helpful, although its mechanism of action is indirect, and occurs through improved vasomotor symptoms and mood disorders (depression) and delays urogenital atrophy.[49,50] No guidelines currently exist for testosterone therapy, but this hormone appears to have a direct role in sexual desire: there is no consensus regarding the definition of 'normal' levels in women, or therapeutic dosage ranges. The known side effects of testosterone in women include decreased levels of high-density lipoprotein, acne, and masculinization. The effects on lipoprotein levels are rarely significant if testosterone is co-administered with estrogen. Patients with a history of breast cancer, uncontrolled hyperlipidemia, liver disease, or hirsutism should not receive testosterone. Lipid levels and liver function tests should be checked every 6 months, and routine Pap smears and mammography should be obtained.

Sexual arousal disorders

These disorders may be due to inadequate stimulation. Encouraging adequate foreplay or the use of vibrators may be helpful. Estrogen replacement therapy may alleviate urogenital atrophy, the most common cause of arousal problems in postmenopausal women. Long-term use of estrogen vaginal creams will require progesterone opposition unless they use the estradiol-containing vaginal ring, Estring. Patients who do not wish to use the ring during the day often achieve sufficient relief with night-time use only. Water-based lubricants may also prove effective. Microvascular disease of the vagina may be a particular problem for diabetic women. A small study with sildenafil in women with type 1 DM improved arousal disorder.[51]

Orgasmic disorders

Anorgasmia is often caused by sexual inexperience or lack of sufficient stimulation. Treatment consists of maximizing stimulation while minimizing inhibition. Stimulation may include masturbation, the use of a vibrator or Kegel exercises. Strategies to minimize inhibition include fantasizing, listening to background music, and videos or 'spectatoring' (watching oneself as if from a third-person perspective).

Sexual pain disorders

For dyspareunia, warm baths and non-steroidal inflammatory medications before intercourse may be helpful. Additionally, the female on top position is preferred for control of penetration. Use of water-based lubricants can be very helpful, and, occasionally, topical lidocaine may be used.

Conclusion

Men and women with diabetes are at increased risk for developing a variety of sexual disorders. They often may not seek treatment due to embarrassment, ignorance, or misinformation. Because of the wide variety of treatment options currently available to manage sexual dysfunction, clinicians must be proactive in inquiring about sexual problems. Clinicians need to feel knowledgeable about and comfortable in discussing sexual problems with their patients. Much research is needed, particularly in the development of medial treatments for female sexual dysfunction.

References

1. Ayta IA, McKinlay JB, Krane RJ. The likely worldwide increase in erectile dysfunction between 1995 and 2025 and some possible policy consequences. BJU Int 1999; 84(1): 50–6.
2. Johannes CB, Araujo AB, Feldman HA et al. Incidence of erectile dysfunction in men 40–69 years old: longitudinal results from the Massachusetts male aging study. J Urol 2000; 163(2): 460–3.
3. Polsky JY, Aronson KJ, Heaton PJ et al. Smoking and other lifestyle factors in relation to erectile dysfunction. BJU Int 2005; 96(9): 1355–9.
4. Feldman HA, Goldstein I, Hatzichristou DG et al. Impotence and its medical and psychosocial correlates: results of the Massachusetts Male Aging Study. J Urol 1994; 151: 54–61.

5. Araujo AB, Durante R, Feldman HA et al. The relationship between depressive symptoms and male erectile dysfunction: cross-sectional results from the Massachusetts Male Aging Study. Psychosom Med 1998; 60: 458–65.

6. Lewis RW. Epidemiology of erectile dysfunction. Urol Clin North Am 2001; 28: 209–16.

7. Fedele D, Coscelli C, Cucinotta D et al. Incidence of erectile dysfunction in Italian men with diabetes. J Urol 2001; 166: 1368–71.

8. Romeo JH, Seftel AD, Madhun ZT et al. Sexual function in men with diabetes type 2: association with glycemic control. J Urol 2000; 163: 788–91.

9. Vickers MA, Wright EA. Erectile dysfunction in the patient with diabetes mellitus. Am J Manag Care 2004; 10(1 Suppl): S3–11.

10. Thase ME, Reynolds CF, Jennings JR et al. Nocturnal penile tumescence is diminished in depressed men. Biol Psychiatry 1988; 24: 33–46.

11. Shabsigh R, Lein LT, Seidman S et al. Increased incidence of depressive symptoms in men with erectile dysfunction. Urology 1998; 52: 848–52.

12. Seidman SN, Roose SP, Menza MA et al. Treatment of erectile dysfunction in men with depressive symptoms: results of a placebo-controlled trial with sildenafil citrate. Am J Psychiatry 2001; 158: 1623–30.

13. Rosen RC, Seidman SN, Menza MA et al. Quality of life, mood and sexual function: a path analytic model of treatment effects in men with erectile dysfunction and depressive symptoms. Int J Impotence Res 2004; 16(4): 334–40.

14. Rosen R, Shabsigh R, Berber M et al. Efficacy and tolerability of vardenafil in men with mild depression and erectile dysfunction: the depression-related improvement with vardenafil for erectile response study. Am J Psychiatry 2006; 163(1): 79–87.

15. Thethi TK, Asafu-Adjaye NO, Fonseca VA. Erectile dysfunction. Clin Diabet 2005; 23(3): 105–13.

16. Yamanaka G, Otsuka K, Hotta N et al. Depressive mood is independently related to stroke and cardiovascular events in a community. Biomed Pharmacother 2005; 59 (Suppl 1): S31–9.

17. Sullivan ME, Keoghane SR, Miller MA. Vascular risk factors and erectile dysfunction. BJU Int 2001; 87: 838–45.

18. El-Sakka A, Tayeb KA. Erectile dysfunction risk factors in noninsulin dependent diabetic Saudi patients. J Urol 2003; 169: 1043–7.

19. Fedele D, Coscelli C, Cucinotta D et al. Incidence of erectile dysfunction in Italian men with diabetes. J Urol 2001; 166: 1368–71.

20. Aizenberg D, Zemishlany Z, Dorfman-Etrog P et al. Sexual dysfunction in male schizophrenic patients. J Clin Psychiatry 1995; 56(4): 137–41.

21. Olfson M, Uttaro T, Carson WH et al. Male sexual dysfunction and quality of life in schizophrenia. J Clin Psychiatry 2005; 66(3): 331–8.

22. Ghadirian AM, Chouinard G, Annable L. Sexual dysfunction and plasma prolactin levels in neuroleptic-treated schizophrenic outpatients. J Nerv Ment Dis 1982; 170 (8): 463–7.

23. Laumann EO, Paik A, Rosen RC. Sexual dysfunction in the United States: prevalence and predictors. JAMA 1999; 281: 537–44.

24. Dunn KM, Croft PR, Hackett GI. Association of sexual problems with social, psychological, and physical problems in men and women: a cross sectional population survey. J Epidemiol Community Health 1999; 53: 144–8.

25. Basson R, Berman J, Burnett A et al. Report of the international consensus development conference on female sexual dysfunction: definitions and classifications. J Urol 2000; 163: 888–93.

26. Rutherford D, Collier A. Sexual dysfunction in women with diabetes mellitus. Gynecol Endocrinol 2005; 21(4): 189–92.
27. Enzlin P, Mathieu C, Van den Bruel A et al. Sexual dysfunction in women with type 1 diabetes: a controlled study. Diabetes Care 2002; 25: 672–7.
28. Schiel R, Muller UA. Prevalence of sexual disorders in a selection-free diabetic population (JEVIN). Diabetes Res Clin Pract 1999; 44: 115–21.
29. Enzlin P, Mathieu C, Van Den Bruel A, Vanderschueren D, Demyttenaere K. Prevalence and predictors of sexual dysfunction in patients with type 1 diabetes. Diabetes Care 2003; 26(2): 409–14.
30. Schreiner-Engel P, Schaivi RC, Viettorisz D, Smith H. The differential impact of diabetes type on female sexuality. J Psychosom Res 1987; 31: 23–33.
31. Moran S. Pathophysiology of diabetic sexual dysfunction. J Endocrinol Invest 2003; 26(3 Suppl): 65–9.
32. Quirk FH, Heiman JR, Rosen RC et al. Development of a sexual function questionnaire for clinical trials of female sexual dysfunction. J Womens Health Gend Based Med 2002; 11(3): 277–89.
33. O'Leary MP, Fowler FJ, Lenderking WR et al. The brief male sexual function inventory for urology. Urology 1995; 46: 697–706.
34. Clayton AH, McGarvey EL, Clavet GJ. The Changes in Sexual Functioning Questionnaire (CSFQ): development, reliability, and validity. Psychopharmacol Bull 1997; 33: 731–45.
35. Mellinger DC. Preparing students with diabetes for life at college. Diabetes Care 2003; 26(9): 2675–8.
36. Nurnberg HG, Hensley PL, Gelenberg AJ et al. Treatment of antidepressant-associate sexual dysfunction with sildenafil: a randomized controlled trial. JAMA 2003; 289(1): 56–64.
37. Fava M, Nurnberg HG, Seidman SN et al. Efficacy and safety of sildenafil in men with serotonergic antidepressant-associated erectile dysfunction: results from a randomized, double-blind, placebo-controlled trial. J Clin Psychiatry 2006; 67(2): 240–6.
38. Jackson G, Gillies H, Osterloh I. Past, present, and future: a 7-year update of Viagra (sildenafil citrate). Int J Clin Pract 2005; 59(6): 680–91.
39. Rendell MS, Rajfer J, Wicker PA et al. Sildenafil for treatment of eretile dysfunction in men with diabetes: a randomized controlled trial. Sildenafil Diabetes Study Group. JAMA 1999; 281(5): 421–6.
40. Bronwyn GA, Stuckey MD, Jadzinsky MN et al. Sildenafil citrate for treatment of erectile dysfunction in men with type 1 diabetes: results of a randomized controlled trial. Diabetes Care 2003; 26: 279–84.
41. Goldstein I, Young JM, Fischer J et al. Vardenafil, a new phosphodiesterase type 5 inhibitor, in the treatment of erectile dysfunction in men with diabetes: a multlicenter double-blind placebo-controlled fixed-dose study. Diabetes Care 2003; 26 (3): 777–83.
42. Saenz de Tejada I, Anglin G, Knight JR et al. Effects of tadalafil on erectile dysfunction in men with diabetes. Diabetes Care 2002; 25(12): 2159–64.
43. Fonseca V, Seftel A, Denne J et al. Impact of diabetes mellitus on the severity of erectile dysfunction and response to treatment: analysis of data from tadalafil clinical trials. Diabetologia 2004; 47(11): 1914–23.
44. Lue TF, Giuliano F, Montorsi F et al. Summary of the recommendations on sexual dysfunctions in men. J Sex Med 2004; 1(1): 6–23.

45. Heaton JPW, Morales A, Adams MA, Johnston B, El-Rashidy R. Recovery of erectile function by the oral administration of apomorphine. Urology 1995; 45(2): 200–6.
46. Bukofzer S, Livesey N. Safety and tolerability of apomorphine SL (Uprima). Int J Impot Res 2001; 13(Suppl 3): S40–4.
47. Basu A, Ryder RE. New treatment options for erectile dysfunction in patients with diabetes mellitus. Drugs 2004; 64(23): 2667–88.
48. Gontero P, D'Antonio R, Pretti G et al. Clinical efficacy of apomorphine SL in erectile dysfunction of diabetic men. Int J Impot Res 2005; 17(1): 80–5.
49. Davis SR, Guay AT, Shifren JL, Mazer NA. Endocrine aspects of female sexual dysfunction. J Sex Med 2004; 1(1): 82–6.
50. Phillips NA. Female sexual dysfunction: evaluation and treatment. Am Fam Physician 2000; 62(1): 127–36.
51. Caruso S, Rugolo S, Agnello C et al. Sildenafil improves sexual functioning in premenopausal women with type 1 diabetes who are affected by sexual arousal disorder: a double-blind, crossover, placebo-controlled pilot study. Fertil Steril 2006; 85(5): 1496–501.

Diabetic peripheral neuropathic pain: an inevitable consequence of diabetes mellitus?

B Eliot Cole and Maria D Llorente

Introduction

Diabetic neuropathy (DN) occurs in 50% of people living with diabetes mellitus (DM), and is the most significant cause of foot ulcers in this population. Although most people with DN will not experience pain, a significant number do, adversely affecting mood, sleep, self-esteem, and quality of life measures, and compromising activities of daily living. There is little consensus regarding the pathophysiologic etiologies of pain, the best diagnostic tools to adequately evaluate patients, and optimal treatment choices to be considered. The numbers of patients suffering with diabetic peripheral neuropathic pain is likely to increase given the current worldwide exponential growth in incidence of diabetes and the increase in life expectancies for diabetic individuals. This chapter addresses the core concepts and evaluation strategies regarding DN and neuropathic pain.

Epidemiology and costs

Diabetic neuropathy is defined as the presence of signs and/or symptoms of peripheral nerve dysfunction in people with diabetes after other causes have been excluded. It is the most common form of neuropathy worldwide. It is generally agreed that a diagnosis of DN should be based on at least two abnormalities, with, ideally, one of these two coming from results of quantitative tests or electrophysiology. In the USA, the prevalence of DN is generally estimated at 50% (range of 10–100%).[1–6] Extrapolating from large-population samples, there may be as many as 7 million US citizens afflicted with DN,[3,7] and, although not all are symptomatic, 27% will experience diabetic peripheral neuropathic pain (DPNP) that will require medical intervention.[8]

DN is implicated in 50–75% of all non-traumatic amputations in the USA.[3–5,9–11] In Western countries, diabetic foot disease is the most common cause of hospitalization among diabetics, who are 15 times more likely than non-diabetics to have amputations.[9–11] Total direct costs for healing infected foot ulcers not requiring amputation were $17 500 (in 1998 US dollars), with the costs for lower-extremity amputations around $30 000 to $33 500, depending on the level of amputation.[12] As the number of persons with diabetes increases worldwide, the projected costs will be staggering.[13] As an example, the total annual cost of DN and its complications in the USA is now estimated to be between $4.6 and $13.7 billion (2001 US dollars).[14]

Classification and clinical symptoms of diabetic neuropathy

Classification of DN at the present time is based on the clinical manifestations (Table 6.1). The three approaches most commonly used are:

- polyneuropathy vs mononeuropathy
- length-dependent (distal, large fibers, and symmetric) vs focal vs non-diabetic neuropathies
- those that are rapidly reversible and asymmetric vs generalized symmetrical vs focal.[8]

Manifestations of disease can range from subclinical to clinical symptoms, depending on the type of nerve fibers involved.[15] Prognostically, sensorimotor polyneuropathies and autonomic neuropathies generally progress with time, whereas mononeuropathies, radiculopathies, and acute painful neuropathies present with severe pain but are short-lived and then generally remit.[16]

The acute painful neuropathy, associated with poor glycemic control, often follows an episode of ketoacidosis, and presents with rapid onset of severe distal burning pain and aching, worse at night and accompanied by sudden weight loss.[8,17]

Table 6.1 Classification of diabetic neuropathy and associated clinical symptoms

	Physical symptoms
Symmetric	
Sensorimotor:	
Distal symmetric polyneuropathy	Sensory nerves: aching, squeezing, freezing, throbbing, and feeling as though walking on marbles, numbness, paresthesia, cramping, burning, pain
	Motor nerves: muscle weakness, inability to stand from a seated position, and spontaneous fasciculations
Acute painful neuropathy	Sudden onset of burning pain, worse at night, with weight loss. Can occur after sudden improvement in glycemic control or following ketoacidosis
Asymmetric	
Focal neuropathy:	
Diabetic mononeuropathy	Somatic:
	Nerve entrapment/compression: may be bilateral, carpal tunnel syndrome
	Ischemia/infarction: acute, focal pain, associated with weakness and variable sensory loss
	Cranial: acute periorbital pain, headache, diplopia, muscle weakness (III, IV, VI), Bell's palsy, ptosis, (VII)
Mononeuropathy multiplex	Multiple nerves affected as above randomly
Truncal neuropathy	Chest/abdominal burning, stabbing, beltlike or aching pain, ↑ at night, unilateral onset, may become bilateral, hyperesthesia, weakness of abdominal muscles and quadriceps (L3–L4 involvement)
Diabetic amyotrophy	Sudden, severe unilateral pain in lower back/hips/anterior thigh, bilateral thigh muscle weakness and atrophy, pain, loss of patellar reflex, significant weight loss

Table 6.1 Continued

	Physical symptoms
Autonomic	
Cardiovascular	Dizziness, fatigue, syncope, exercise intolerance, limb hair loss
Gastrointestinal	Diarrhea, constipation, fecal incontinence, dysphagia, bloating, vomiting of retained food, delayed gastric emptying
Endocrine	Lack of awareness of hypoglycemia
Genitourinary	Decreased libido, erectile dysfunction, decreased arousal, anorgasmia, dyspareunia, loss of bladder control, urinary tract infections
Sudomotor	Pruritis, dry skin, $\downarrow$ sweating, $\uparrow$ sweating in defined areas
Ophthalmic	$\downarrow$ dark adaptation, sensitivity to bright lights

Data from [8,15,16,20]

Focal and multifocal neuropathies seen in DN typically appear acutely, are more associated with type 2 DM than type 1 DM, have a weaker association with hyperglycemia than the symmetric neuropathies, and may be associated with inflammatory angiitis and ischemia. The somatic mononeuropathies are typically caused by nerve entrapment or compression, or are a result of infarction of the nerve due to ischemia. Carpal tunnel syndrome (median nerve entrapment) is the most common focal neuropathy seen in diabetics, followed by ulnar entrapment at the elbow. Compression of the lateral femoral cutaneous nerve results in pain, paresthesias, and sensory loss in the lateral thigh. Obesity is its most common cause, followed by trauma, rather than diabetes per se.[8] Focal cranial neuropathies in diabetic patients are rarely seen, occur in older patients with longer disease duration, and primarily affect cranial nerves III, IV, VI and VII. These neuropathies typically recover spontaneously in 3–6 months, but may recur. Optimizing glycemic control and minimizing ischemia, hypertension, and hyperlipidemia may aid in recovery.[8]

Focal truncal neuropathies are mainly seen in middle-aged to elderly type 2 diabetic men.[8] Symptom onset is usually acute, asymmetric, and sensory deficits are in a dermatomal distribution. Symptoms can extend to the neck, lower back, or the contralateral side, but may resolve spontaneously within 3–12 months, although some symptoms may persist and progress in certain persons.

Diabetic amyotrophy is usually bilateral, and often associated with significant weight loss. It, too, occurs with increased frequency in older men with poorly controlled type 2 DM. Symptoms start unilaterally, but can spread to the contralateral side. The thigh muscles (iliopsoas, quadriceps, and adductors) atrophy, causing weakness, occasionally pain, and loss of patellar reflexes. Recovery is often spontaneous, within 6–12 months, but may recur.

Symptoms of autonomic dysregulation can be found in up to 50% of patients with diabetes. These symptoms are classified based on the organ system affected (see Table 6.1)[18] and are often the presenting complaint to a variety of specialists. Cardiac autonomic neuropathy (CAN) may lead to arrhythmia without cardiac ischemia.[19]

Chronic sensorimotor distal symmetric neuropathy, what is commonly thought of as diabetic peripheral neuropathy (DPN), is the most frequent form of neuropathy associated with DM. Many patients are asymptomatic and only present for medical care due to painless foot ulceration. The longest peripheral nerves are affected first, with sensory, motor, and autonomic functioning affected differentially. Sensory dysfunction is usually most prominent.

Those who develop diabetic neuropathic pain often describe bilateral burning, muscle cramps, lancinating (piercing or stabbing) pain, electrical sensations, hyperalgesia (exaggerated pain sensation to normally painful stimuli), and allodynia (pain with normally non-painful innocuous stimuli). Traditionally, these symptoms begin and are worse in the feet and are more likely to occur at night. Gradual ascending progression occurs in a stocking pattern. Once symptoms reach the knees, the hands begin to develop similar symptoms in a glove distribution. As smaller nerve fibers become involved, pain and temperature sensation is lost, and at this point, the individual is now predisposed to the development of foot ulcers. Because of proprioceptive loss, unsteadiness can develop, often leading to fall-related trauma.[8] Table 6.2 describes the differential diagnosis of a variety of painful disease processes that may also affect patients with DM, but have clinical features that distinguish them from DPNP, and should be ruled out. The remainder of this chapter will focus on DPN.

Staging the severity of diabetic neuropathy

An Expert Consensus Panel developed guidelines for clinical staging of DPN severity for use in clinical practice, clinical trials, and epidemiologic studies as follows:

- *Stage 0* (no neuropathy): no symptoms and fewer than two abnormalities on testing (nerve conduction velocity [NCV], neurologic examination, threshold of vibration, cooling or warming sensation, or autonomic function).
- *Stage 1* (symptomatic neuropathy): no symptoms and two or more abnormalities on functional testing.
- *Stage 2:* symptoms of a lesser degree than stage 3 and two or more functional abnormalities.
- *Stage 3* (disabling neuropathy): disabling symptoms and two or more functional abnormalities.[20]

Table 6.2   Differential diagnosis of neuropathy signs and symptoms in patients with diabetes

Disease process	Distinguishing features
Claudication	Intermittent, lower extremity pain that worsens with walking and is relieved with rest
Morton's neuroma	Unilateral pain, more often seen in women, elicited by thumb pressure on between the 1st and 4th metatarsal heads
Osteoarthritis	Early morning stiffness, diminished joint motion, flexion contractures may be present, pain worsens with exercise and improves with rest
Charcot's neuroarthropathy	Pain associated with increased blood flow due to heating of foot, ↓ warm sensory perception, vibratory sense loss
Plantar fasciitis	Shooting/burning pain in heel with walking, worse with prolonged activity, tenderness in plantar region upon ankle dorsiflexion
Tarsal tunnel syndrome	Pain and numbness radiating from medial malleolus to sole, entrapment of posterior tibial nerve
Erythromelalgia	Burning pain and erythema of toes, forefoot and hands, associated with ambient temperature change so patients avoid wearing socks; pain relieved by walking on cold surfaces, soaking in cold water, rest, and elevation of legs
Vitamin B_{12} deficiency	Paresthesias, vibratory sense loss, imbalance, low serum vitamin B_{12} levels

Data from[3]

Understanding the pathophysiology of diabetic neuropathy

The pathophysiologic etiology of DPN is incompletely understood, but several hypotheses have been investigated.[21] Diabetes is a hypermetabolic state that results in elevated intracellular glucose levels. Interestingly, whether DPN develops is not related to glycemic control. The overall severity and progression of neuropathy, however, is related.[3,22,23] For example, impaired glucose tolerance (IGT) is associated with a milder form of neuropathy than that seen in patients with diabetes.[24] In type 1 DM, the most rapid nerve function deterioration occurs soon after disease onset and, within 2–3 years, the process slows down. In type 2 DM, NCV slowing may be present at diagnosis, and then progresses over time.

Elevated intracellular glucose levels saturate the normal glycolytic pathway, activating the polyol pathway, an alternative catabolic form of glucose metabolism. The first step of the polyol pathway is the conversion of glucose to sorbitol and then fructose. The rate-limiting enzyme is aldose reductase. Among patients with type 2 DM, those with higher set points for aldose reductase activity were more likely to develop DPN. It is believed that accumulation of sorbitol and fructose leads to depletion of glutathione and the accumulation of toxic metabolites, oxidative stress, increased production of advanced glycation end-products (AGEs), and activation of diacylglycerol and protein kinase C (PKC).[21] AGEs induce monocytes and endothelial cells to increase production of cytokines and adhesion molecules,[25] which can lead to capillary damage and decreased perfusion, slowing of axonal transport, and eventually, nerve degeneration.

The mechanisms leading to neuropathic pain include central sensitization, reduced inhibition, sympathetic activation, and peripheral sensitization. *Central sensitization* involves hypersensitivity of dorsal horn neurons, lowered threshold for activation, expanded receptor fields, and activation of excitatory neurotransmitters and N-methyl-D-aspartate (NMDA) receptors resulting in intracellular calcium accumulation. *Reduced inhibition* in the brainstem's descending pathways is modulated by endorphins, serotonin, and norepinephrine, leading to disinhibition and further perpetuation of the centrally mediated pain. *Sympathetic activation* is induced as the injured nerve then activates sympathetic nerve endings to sprout from nearby blood vessels, enhancing signal transmission to the dorsal root ganglion, which can cause sympathetically mediated pain. Lastly, *peripheral sensitization* occurs as nerve injury may lead to hyperexcitability of peripheral nerve nociceptors and further transduction of painful stimuli.[26]

Clinical assessment of diabetic neuropathy

Many patients with DPN are asymptomatic and deficits may be identified during a routine neurological examination. Those who are symptomatic often have difficulty describing the symptoms of DPN. Pain is a very personal experience, and there may be significant variations in patient reports with similar degrees of physical findings. Additionally, symptoms of neuropathy may not be DPN, and other etiologies for symptoms should be considered.

Risk factors

A number of factors have been identified that are associated with an increased risk for DPN, and should be part of an initial evaluation, including:

- personal factors (older age, greater weight, taller height)
- diabetes-related factors (longer duration of diabetes, history of poorly controlled glycemia and ketoacidosis, increased hemoglobin A1c [HbA$_{1c}$] levels)
- vascular factors (hypertension, hypertriglyceridemia, decreased high-density lipoprotein [HDL] cholesterol). Tobacco use has been found to be a risk factor in some, but not all, studies.

Descriptive, numeric, and visual pain scales

Commonly used tools to assess pain intensity include:

- *descriptive* words (none, mild, moderate, severe, overwhelming, incapacitating, worst possible) in the Descriptive Rating Scale (DRS)
- *numeric* anchors (0–10, with 0 signifying no pain and 10 the worst pain possible or imagined) for the Numeric Rating Scale (NRS)
- an open-ended *Visual* Analog Scale (VAS) with only the terms 'no pain' and 'worst pain' as end-point anchors.

The choice of a particular scale is determined by the patients served (children vs adults, English speakers vs non-English speakers), the clinical environment, and familiarity of practitioners with the scales.

As a matter of practitioner convenience and efficiency, many patients are simply asked to rate their pain intensity verbally between 0 and 10. Although the use of one of the actual rating scales is theoretically more reliable and is necessary for conducting clinical studies, just quantifying the pain intensity at each point of contact leads to common ground between patients and providers and ultimately better therapy. Failure to monitor the intensity of pain objectively makes comparison of therapeutic efforts unreliable, and, relative to prescribing opioid therapy, may even lead to disciplinary sanctions by professional boards.

DPN-specific screening instruments

Several screening questionnaires are available to assess the quality, location, and severity of DPN symptoms with varying degrees of sensitivity and specificity.[27–31] It is well-recognized that the pain, symptoms, and deficits associated with DPN have significant adverse effects on quality of life and mood. Clinicians should inquire about the impact of the symptoms on the person's daily functioning, and all patients with diabetes should be screened at least annually for depression.

Physical examination

The neurologic examination of the lower extremities is the most important component of the clinical diagnosis of DPN. Key sensory domains to evaluate include pressure, vibration, temperature, and pin prick. Vibration sense is tested by application of a 128 Hz tuning fork to the great toe. Vibratory sense is intact if the patient feels the vibration. Pressure sensation is assessed using a $10g$ (the force needed to buckle) Semmes–Weinstein monofilament. The filament is gently applied to the 1st, 3rd, and 5th hallux and metatarsal heads just until the nylon filament buckles. If not detected the patient is at risk of foot ulceration.[8] Test tubes of warm or cold water placed against the dorsum of the foot establish the presence (if felt) or absence (if not felt) of temperature sensation. Pin prick sensation is assessed by applying just enough pressure to deform the skin; this is often done in conjunction with dull/blunt sensation. Patients should be able to differentiate between sharp and dull pain easily, so any loss of discrimination is diagnostic.

Laboratory investigations

Baseline serum laboratories should include glycosylated hemoglobin A_{1c} (HbA_{1c}), comprehensive metabolic panel (including renal and hepatic function tests), thyroid function tests, and vitamin B_{12} levels. Because of the frequent co-occurrence of DN, knowing current renal function is needed for appropriate use of renally excreted medications (gabapentin and pregabalin) and metabolites (opioids). With opioids in particular, elimination involves hepatic metabolism and then urinary excretion of metabolites. In the presence of adequate liver function, but poor renal excretion, accumulation of potentially antianalgesic substances (morphine-3-glucuronide) can counteract analgesic effects. Similarly, the accumulation of central nervous system toxic opioid metabolites (morphine-3-glucuronide, normorphine, normeperidine) can cause confusion, delirium, myoclonus, and seizures.

Electrodiagnostics

Nerve conduction studies (NCS) measure speed (velocity of impulses), amplitude (number of nerve fibers capable of conducting impulses), and shape of neurologic response in order to detect demyelination and axon loss. NCS are routinely performed with electromyograms (EMGs), a measure of the electrical activity of muscles. NCS are objective, valid, and reproducible, and are the most useful electrodiagnostic indicator for DPN.[32] NCS provide a sensitive yet non-specific index of DPN that may be used to track the progression of DPN as well as its response to improved glycemic control.[8] F-wave testing is a type of NCS performed on motor nerves more proximal to the spine. This type of testing is useful in diagnosing radiculopathies, plexopathies, and proximal mononeuropathies. There is no correlation between NCS results, however, and severity of pain symptoms.

Psychiatric comorbidities

There are several reasons to screen all patients with DPN for psychiatric comorbidities. First, several psychiatric disorders have been identified as independent risk factors for the development of type 2 DM, most notably schizophrenia and depression.[33,34] Secondly, having a psychiatric disorder is associated with an increased risk of poorer glycemic control, and greater number and severity of diabetes complications, including the development of DPN.[35,36] Thirdly, diabetes itself is a difficult illness with which to cope. More than 90% of the management of this illness is on the shoulders of the patient. Diabetes often requires major behavioral lifestyle changes. Patients face the possibility of chronic and disabling complications including sexual dysfunction, loss of vision, and amputation. Additionally, patients with DPNP may also be at increased risk for committing suicide due to the co-occurrence of unrecognized psychiatric illness (such as depression) and inadequately managed pain.[37] They have many resources available to end their lives, including insulin, narcotics, and tricyclic antidepressants. Most importantly, studies have suggested that successful treatment for both schizophrenia and diabetes may have favorable effects on glucose regulation. These effects could potentially delay the development and/or progression of DPN and the associated pain.

Patient and family education

To improve diabetes outcomes and diabetes self-management, the patient and his family need to have an adequate understanding of DPN. The core educational intervention should include:

- a basic understanding of the underlying basis of neuropathic pain
- the important role of glycemic control in the prevention of progression of neuropathy
- realistic expectations of what can be achieved with currently available treatment options
- how pain flare ups are to be managed
- who will be the primary provider responsible for pain management.

Summary

DNP is a highly prevalent condition, and its etiology is likely associated with poorer glycemic control. Many patients will be asymptomatic, but with physical findings on neurologic examination. Other patients will experience a variety of symptoms, ranging from uncomfortable to painful to disabling pain. Management of DPN begins with a thorough assessment and examination, and should include electrodiagnostics to be able to adequately stage the degree of pathology. Patients should also be screened for underlying psychiatric conditions, and if identified, referred for treatment. Each practitioner working with diabetic patients plays an important role and must provide emotional support. This includes reinforcing the importance of optimal glycemic control, the need for daily or twice-daily foot care, and encouraging faithful adherence to treatment. The presence of this chronic disease is burdensome, unpleasant, and life-altering for patients. High-quality patient care enlists the patient as a collaborator in assessing and describing symptoms relating response to management options.

References

1. Vinik AI, Mitchell BD, Leichter SB et al. Epidemiology of the complications of diabetes. In: Leslie RDG, Robbins DC, eds. Diabetes: Clinical Science in Practice. Cambridge, UK: Cambridge University Press, 1994: 221–87.
2. Dyck PJ, Kratz KM, Karnes JL et al. The prevalence by staged severity of various types of diabetic neuropathy, retinopathy, and nephropathy in a population-based cohort: the Rochester Diabetic Neuropathy Study. Neurology 1993; 43: 817–24.
3. Vinik AI, Mehrabyan A. Diabetic neuropathies. Med Clin North Am 2004; 88: 947–99.
4. Holzer SE, Camerota A, Martens L et al. Costs and duration of care for lower extremity ulcers in patients with diabetes. Clin Ther 1998; 20: 169–81.
5. Caputo GM, Cavanagh PR, Ulbrecht JS, Gibbons GW, Karchmer AW. Assessment and management of foot disease in patients with diabetes. N Engl J Med 1994; 331: 854–60.
6. Young MJ, Boulton AJM, MacLeod AF, Williams DRR, Sonksen PH. A multicentre study of the prevalence of diabetic peripheral neuropathy in the United Kingdom hospital clinic population. Diabetologia 1993; 36: 1–5.
7. Pirart J. Diabetes mellitus and its degenerative complications: a prospective study of 4,400 patients observed between 1947 and 1973 (3rd and last part). Diabetes Metab 1977; 3: 245–56.
8. Boulton AJM, Malik RA, Arezzo JC, Sosenko JM. Diabetic somatic neuropathies. Diabetes Care 2004; 27: 1458–86.
9. Most RS, Sinnock P. The epidemiology of lower limb extremity amputations in diabetic individuals. Diabetes Care 1983; 6: 87–91.
10. Trautner C, Haastert B, Giani G, Berger M. Incidence of lower limb amputations and diabetes. Diabetes Care 1996; 19: 1006–9.
11. Morris AD, McAlpine R, Steinke D et al. for the DARTS/MEMO Collaboration. Diabetes and lower-limb amputations in the community: a retrospective cohort study. Diabetes Care 1998; 21: 738–43.
12. Tennvall GR, Apelqvist J. Health-economic consequences of diabetic foot lesions. Clin Infect Dis 2004; 39: S132–9.
13. Thomas PK. Diabetic peripheral neuropathies: their cost to patient and society and the value of knowledge of risk factors for development of interventions. Eur Neurol 1999; 41: 35–43.
14. Gordois A, Scuffham P, Shearer A, Oglesby A, Tobian JA. The health care costs of diabetic peripheral neuropathy in the US. Diabetes Care 2003; 26: 1790–5.
15. Boulton AJM, Vinik AI, Arezzo JC et al. Diabetic neuropathies: a statement by the American Diabetes Association. Diabetes Care 2005; 28(4): 956–62.
16. Watkins PJ. Progression of diabetic autonomic neuropathy. Diabet Med 1993; 10(Suppl 2): 77–8S.
17. Boulton AJM. Management of diabetic peripheral neuropathy. Clin Diabetes 2005; 23: 9–15. Available at: http://clinical.diabetesjournals.org/cgi/content/abstract/23/1/9. Accessed on 1/17/2006.
18. National Institutes of Health (NIH). Diabetes among older adults imposed an estimated $133.5 billion cost in 1990s. Available at: http://www.nih.gov/news/pr/nov 2004/nia-15.htm Accessed on 1/18/2006.
19. Bloomgarden ZT. Diabetic retinopathy and neuropathy. Diabetes Care 2005; 28: 963–70.

20. Dyck PJ. Detection, characterization, and staging of polyneuropathy: assessed in diabetes. Muscle Nerve 1988; 11: 21–32.

21. Duby JJ, Campbell RK, Setter SM, White JR, Rasmussen KA. Diabetic neuropathy: an intensive review. Am J Health Syst Pharm 2004; 61: 160–76.

22. Dyck PJ, Davies JL, Wilson DM et al. Risk factors for severity of diabetic polyneuropathy: intensive longitudinal assessment of the Rochester Diabetic Neuropathy Study cohort. Diabetes Care 1999; 22: 1479–86.

23. Partanen J, Niskanen L, Lehtinen J et al. Natural history of peripheral neuropathy in patients with non-insulin dependent diabetes. N Engl J Med 1995; 333: 89–94.

24. Sundkvist G, Dahlin LB, Nilsson H et al. Sorbitol and myo-inositol levels and morphology of sural nerve in relation to peripheral nerve function and clinical neuropathy in men with diabetic, impaired, and normal glucose tolerance. Diabet Med 2000; 17: 259–68.

25. King RH. The role of glycation in the pathogenesis of diabetic polyneuropathy. Mol Pathol 2001; 54: 400–8.

26. Chen H, Lamer TJ, Rho RH et al. Contemporary management of neuropathic pain for the primary care physician. Mayo Clin Proc 2004; 79: 1533–45.

27. Zelman DC, Dukes E, Brandenburg N, Bostrom A, Gore M. Identification of cut-points for mild, moderate and severe pain due to diabetic peripheral neuropathy. Pain 2005; 115: 29–36.

28. Jensen MP, Friedman M, Bonzo D, Richards P. The validity of the Neuropathic Pain Scale for assessing diabetic neuropathic pain in a clinical trial. Clin J Pain 2006; 22: 97–103.

29. Backonja M-M, Krause SJ. Neuropathic Pain Questionnaire-Short Form. Clin J Pain 2003; 19: 315–16.

30. Bennett M. The LANSS Pain Scale: the Leeds assessment of neuropathic symptoms and signs. Pain 2001; 92: 147–57.

31. Bouhassia D, Attal N, Fermanian J et al. Development and validation of the Neuropathic Pain Symptom Inventory. Pain 2004; 108: 248–57.

32. Herrmann DN, Fregusson MI, Logigian EL. Conduction slowing in diabetic distal polyneuropathy. Muscle Nerve 2002; 26: 232–7.

33. Freedland KE. Section II: Hypothesis 1: Depression is a risk factor for the development of type 2 diabetes. Diabetes Spectrum 2004; 17: 150–2.

34. Expert Group. Schizophrenia and Diabetes 2003: Expert Consensus Meeting, Dublin 3–4 October 2003: consensus summary. Br J Psychiatry Suppl 2004; 47: S112–14.

35. de Groot M, Anderson RJ, Freedland KE, Clouse RE, Lustman PJ. Association of depression and diabetes complications: a meta-analysis. Psychosom Med 2001; 63: 619–30.

36. Dixon L, Weiden P, Delahanty J et al. Prevalence and correlates of diabetes in national schizophrenia samples. Schizophr Bull 2000; 26: 903–12.

37. Walsh SM, Sage RA. Depression and chronic diabetic foot disability. A case report of suicide. Clin Podiatr Med Surg 2002; 19(4): 493–508.

HIV-1 infection, diabetes mellitus, and psychiatric disorders

Karl Goodkin, Stephen Symes, Mauricio Concha, Michael Kolber, Deshratn Asthana, Rebeca Molina, Alicia Frasca, Wenli Zheng, Sandra O'Mellan, and Maria del Carmen Lichtenberger

Introduction to diabetes mellitus in the setting of HIV-1 infection

Adult-onset (type 2) diabetes mellitus (DM) has become an increasing concern in the field of HIV/AIDS since the introduction of highly active antiretroviral therapy (HAART), now referred to as combination anti-retroviral therapy (CART), in 1996. The increased incidence of DM has occurred as a long-term toxic side effect of the use of two classes of antiretroviral (ARV) agents – the protease inhibitors (PIs) and the nucle-oside reverse transcriptase inhibitors (nRTIs), predominantly the former. However, it is also thought that the prevalence of metabolic syndrome (characterized by central obesity, dyslipidemia, hypertension, and insulin resistance) associated with DM outside of HIV-1 infection increases in prevalence in the setting of HIV-1 infection. We will examine in this chapter how the risks for DM in the general population interact with those in HIV-1-infected individuals to produce a higher risk for DM and its associated complications of coronary artery disease (CAD), myocardial infarction (MI), and cerebrovascular accident (CVA). We will then exam-ine how neuropsychiatric disorders and treatments common in HIV-1 infection may play a role in the development and treatment of type 2 DM. Finally, we will examine the specific recommendations for neuropsychiatric treatment in the setting of HIV-1 infection complicated by type 2 DM.

Diabetes mellitus risk factors in the general population

Non-modifiable diabetes mellitus risk factors

Older age

Heart disease and CVA are the first and third causes of death, overall, in the USA. The risk for vascular disease increases significantly with age, and the population >50 years old is at a substantially higher risk. In the area of HIV/AIDS, the Centers for Disease Control and Prevention (CDC) have defined 'older age' as ≥50 years old. The number of persons living with AIDS in the USA in the >50-year-old age range increased from 59 649 in 2000 to 112 147 in 2004 – nearly two-fold, with approximately equal increases throughout this age range.[1] The cumulative number of AIDS cases over 50 years old increases, consecutively, from the national level (11%), to the state of Florida (15%), to Miami-Dade County (16.4%).[2] As noted above, the success of CART has reduced morbidity and mortality due to immunosuppression in the short term, but CART has simultaneously increased the risk for such morbidity and mortality in the long term. The predominant reason for this increased long term risk is that of the overlap between age-associated and HIV/AIDS treatment-associated risks for heart disease and CVA.[3]

Ethnicity

It is well known that African and Hispanic Americans share a higher risk of type 2 DM than Caucasian Americans. One study focused on the severe complication of lower-extremity amputations. That study showed that in six metropolitan areas in south Texas, Hispanic Americans (Mexicans) and African Americans had more diabetes-related amputations than Caucasian Americans (86% and 75% versus 56% respectively).[4] Likewise, African American and Hispanic Americans have a higher prevalence of HIV/AIDS than Caucasian Americans. Although Native Americans do not show a high cumulative case burden of HIV/AIDS, they do have a particularly high risk for DM (with the exception of the Inuit).[5] Thus, the screening concerns for DM among African, Hispanic, and non-Inuit Native Americans with HIV/AIDS are yet higher than the already significant concern in the general population.

Family history

Family history, like ethnicity, is well known to be associated with the risk for type 2 DM. As an example, one recent study evaluated the use of self-reported family medical history as a potential screening tool to identify risk for DM in a survey of 4345 US adults. Three family history risk levels were identified, using number and type of affected relatives.

Those with moderate or high family history risk of DM were more likely to report DM (adjusted odds ratio [OR] = 3.6), higher perceived risk for DM (adjusted OR = 4.6), and making lifestyle changes to prevent DM (adjusted OR = 2.2).[6] Positive family history risk for DM identified 73% of all those with DM. As family history of DM was not only associated with having the disease but also with risk awareness and risk-reducing behaviors, screening for family history may also be of utility in the setting of HIV-1 infection. However, in HIV-1 infection there are a number of acquired risk factors other than those described in the general population upon which the impact of family history may, at least in part, be based. These include the presence of lipodystrophy syndrome, the use of a PI and/or nRTI medication, and hepatitis C virus (HCV) co-infection. Hence, family history screening would be expected to be less useful (though still important) as an independent screening technique for DM in the HIV-1-infected population than among the general population.

Other clinical conditions associated with insulin resistance (acanthosis nigricans and polycystic ovary syndrome)

A number of clinical conditions are also known to represent a DM risk. For example, acanthosis nigricans – a condition characterized by hyperplastic lesions affecting localized areas of the skin in persons with obesity and/or hyperinsulinemia – is associated with DM. It involves roughening and darkening of the skin. The presence of this skin lesion has been suggested to be a clinical surrogate of laboratory-documented hyperinsulinemia.[7] Another clinical condition, polycystic ovary syndrome, is likewise associated with DM risk. Polycystic ovary syndrome affects 5–10% of premenopausal women and is one of the most common endocrinopathies of women. It is associated with obesity, amenorrhea, hirsutism, acne, and infertility. By age 40 years, as many as 40% of women with this syndrome will have type 2 DM or impaired glucose tolerance. Furthermore, acanthosis nigricans and polycystic ovary syndrome overlap. A study of Asian women with polycystic ovary syndrome showed that those with acanthosis nigricans had significantly higher body mass indices (BMIs), waist–hip ratios, and prevalence of abnormal glucose tolerance compared with those without acanthosis nigricans.[8] Acanthosis nigricans and waist–hip ratio were independent predictors for abnormal glucose tolerance. Thus, the presence of acanthosis nigricans and (for women) polycystic ovary syndrome in HIV-1-infected individuals should raise the concern to screen for DM.

Modifiable diabetes mellitus risk factors

Weight

Increased adiposity is the most important risk factor in the prevention of type 2 DM. One study of women showed a relative risk of 38.8 for a BMI (weight in kilograms divided by height in meters squared) $\geq 35\,kg/m^2$ and 20.1 for 30.0–$34.9\,kg/m^2$, compared with those with a BMI $<23\,kg/m^2$.[9] The Women's Health Study reported a relative risk for type 2 DM of 3.22 for being overweight and 9.06 for obesity.[10] Similar results have been reported for men.[11] As expected, significant reductions in DM risk have been reported, with interventions aimed to reduce BMI.

In contrast with the issue in the general population of being overweight, the clinical concern with total body weight in HIV-1 infection typically relates to reduced weight or wasting. Although the concern for lower-than-normal body weight has decreased significantly in the CART era, it nevertheless remains as the greater concern than being overweight. Thus, a major difference in the management of DM risk in the HIV-1-infected individual is that weight reduction interventions do not constitute a commensurate focus. However, it should be noted that weight gain in adults shows a relatively narrow window before significant increases occur in DM risk, changing on a kilogram by kilogram basis. Thus, weight reduction programs should be considered for HIV-1 seropositive individuals in whom it is indicated.

Pregnancy and gestational diabetes

A history of gestational diabetes is a known risk factor for subsequent type 2 DM. While many may consider this fact to be irrelevant to the HIV-1-infected woman and her partner, this is no longer the case. With the vertical transmission of HIV-1 stemmed to very low frequencies in the CART era, ethical considerations about pregnancy in HIV-1 infection have been revised – as per the Americans with Disabilities Act (ADA) – such that discouraging pregnancy and/or withholding fertility services based upon HIV-1 serostatus would probably now be unlawful under most circumstances.[12] The reported prevalence of gestational diabetes averages 2–5% in the USA and is typically diagnosed at 6 months but can develop earlier, especially in women at prior risk for DM. Risk factors for gestational diabetes are similar to those for DM and include a prior infant weighing >9 lb (>4 kg) at birth, prior abortion at term or birth defects, a history of frequent miscarriages, and a maternal age over 25 years old. However, as many as 50% of women diagnosed with gestational diabetes have no known risk factors.

Prompt diagnosis is important, as gestational diabetes generates several risks to mother and infant. The infant may be macrosomic, posing a risk of trauma during delivery, hypoglycemia and severe respiratory problems after birth, as well as long-term obesity and glucose intolerance. Postpartum, the pregnancy-induced demand on the mother for greater insulin production (by about 50%) will revert to normal, resulting in euglycemia in nearly all patients, although patients should be screened for DM annually thereafter. Approximately 60% of women who have had gestational diabetes will eventually develop overt type 2 DM. Most women can be treated effectively with diet (to achieve appropriate weight) and exercise, although insulin may be required if euglycemia is not established within 2 weeks. Breast-feeding may be recommended to reduce the infant's DM risk.

Regarding HIV-1 seropositive status in pregnancy, there is little to no systematic published data regarding the issue of gestational diabetes. Given the prevalence of lipodystrophy syndrome with dyslipidemia, ARV medication toxicity associated with insulin resistance, and HCV–HIV-1 co-infection, it might be expected that screening and prompt, effective treatment of gestational diabetes as well as monitoring for the appearance of type 2 DM postpartum is yet more important among HIV-1-seropositive women. Breast-feeding would not be recommended, as it increases the risk for HIV-1 transmission.

Hypertension

Hypertension is a frequent comorbidity with type 2 DM, affecting 20–60% and having a prevalence 1.5–3 times greater than that of age-matched controls. It is not proven to be an independent risk factor for DM, with the exception of the association of DM with the metabolic syndrome in which hypertension is one of the characteristics. As a case in point of the latter, a recent study of 420 consecutively referred patients with essential hypertension excluding known DM were shown to have abnormal glucose metabolism in 68.5%, isolated insulin resistance in 9.3%, impaired fasting glucose in 11.2%, and impaired glucose tolerance in 22.5%.[13] This study also assessed National Cholesterol Education Program (NCEP) Adult Treatment Program (ATP) III panel-defined metabolic syndrome defined by three or more of the following:

- increased waist circumference (> 40 inches for men, > 35 inches for women)
- elevated triglyceride level (≥ 150 mg/dl)
- low high-density lipoprotein (HDL) cholesterol level (< 40 mg/dl in men, < 50 mg/dl in women)
- hypertension (≥ 130/≥ 85 mmHg)
- impaired fasting glucose level (≥ 110 mg/dl).

The frequency of metabolic syndrome by these criteria was 47.9%. The high rate of abnormal glucose metabolism among patients with essential hypertension suggests the possibility of a pathophysiologic linkage, although the negative effects of diuretics and β-blockers on glucose metabolism must also be considered. Regardless, hypertension in association with metabolic syndrome is a highly significant risk factor for DM.

Regarding the interaction with HIV-1 infection, no evidence demonstrates that HIV-1 infection causes hypertension. Whereas HIV-1-associated nephropathy may occur in about 6% of cases, it is not usually associated with hypertension – although it does cause end-stage renal disease. Given the high prevalence of lipodystrophy syndrome associated with features of the metabolic syndrome in the HIV-1-infected individual, it would be expected that hypertension in this setting translates into a risk for DM and that its treatment relates to a reduction of that risk. Dietary changes, weight reduction, salt restriction, exercise, and reduced alcohol consumption are useful interventions for hypertension risk reduction, as the first line of medical treatment.

Lipid levels

Lipid elevations are considered to be a known contributor to the risk for type II DM independent of serum glucose levels. A recent study of type II DM risk in young men with normal fasting glucose levels reported on 208 incident DM cases with fasting plasma glucose levels < 100 mg/dl.[14] In a multivariate model, controlling for age, family history of DM, BMI, physical activity level, smoking status, and fasting plasma glucose level, a serum triglyceride level of > 150 mg/dl was associated with increased DM risk (across all categories of fasting glucose level).

Many also accept that increased low-density lipoprotein (LDL) cholesterol and decreased HDL cholesterol levels are independent risk factors for type 2 DM. One study of middle-aged British men attempted to determine the risk factors for non-insulin-dependent DM in a prospective design with 7735 men aged 40–59 years old.[15] Known and probable cases of DM were excluded. Of the 194 doctor-diagnosed DM cases occurring over the following 12.8 years, higher HDL cholesterol was associated with a decreased relative risk for DM, with an age-adjusted multivariate relative risk of 0.7 (although BMI was the dominant risk at 7.3). Results from another prospective epidemiologic cohort study conducted in Italy involving 1441 randomly selected subjects, ages 14–84 years old and followed over 8 years, showed no effect of HDL on DM incidence.[16] Likewise, there was no effect for age, triglyceride level, blood pressure, combined occupational and leisure physical activity, and total energy intake observed in that sample. Although age had appeared to be a significant DM predictor when studied alone, it was not after adjustment for baseline BMI and/or fasting plasma glucose level. These results emphasize the interplay among DM risk factors and suggest that the lipid profile, in and of itself, may not be the most important of the DM predictors across samples.

Regarding elevated lipid profiles and DM risk in the HIV-1-infected individual, elevated triglyceride levels were described pre-CART in relation to HIV-1 disease progression and associated increases in interferon-α levels.[17] However, in the CART era, the DM risk related to the lipid profile in HIV-1 infection appears to be related to lipodystrophy syndrome associated with dyslipidemia, which is discussed below.

Smoking

Cigarette smoking is often discussed as a risk for DM but is not consistently included in such studies. When included, statistical power is commonly not sufficient to demonstrate its effect. One prospective study of DM focused upon the role of cigarette smoking and examined a Finnish sample of 41 372 participants aged 25–64 years without a history of DM, coronary heart disease, or CVA at baseline. Data on incident DM cases were ascertained through a nationwide data bank.[18] During a mean follow-up period of 21 years, 2770 subjects were diagnosed with DM. Smoking showed an association with DM, controlling for age, study year, education, BMI, systolic blood pressure, physical activity, and coffee and alcohol drinking. The relative risk was 1.57 amongst men smoking a pack a day or more, with a corresponding hazard ratio of 1.87 among women. Smoking increased the risk of type 2 DM at all levels of BMI and physical activity. Hence, though less well studied than other DM risk factors, cigarette smoking may pose a modest, independent DM risk.

HIV-1-seropositive individuals have higher rates of cigarette smoking than the general population, with rates over 70% documented.[19] As with the active management of lipid levels, smoking cessation was not considered a significant issue for intervention pre-CART. Yet smoking cessation decreases the DM risk to close to that in non-smokers, although the risk does remain elevated after 10 years of nicotine abstinence. Smoking cessation programs are known to increase insulin sensitivity and improve lipid profiles. Moreover, the modest weight gain associated with smoking cessation may also reflect an improvement in the health of many HIV-1-seropositive individuals impacted by loss of appetite/weight associated with HIV-1 disease progression. Thus, in the CART era, the HIV-1-seropositive smoker should be referred to smoking cessation programs routinely – to reduce not only DM risk but also other smoking-related health risks.

Physical activity

Physical activity and exercise have been studied relatively frequently as a lifestyle issue related to DM risk. In the Finnish study described above, men engaged in moderate levels of physical activity had a substantially reduced DM risk, relative to physically inactive men – after adjustment for age and BMI – an association which persisted in multivariate analysis.[18] A recent review reported that cross-sectional and retrospective epidemiologic studies provide evidence that lack of physical activity is an independent risk factor for insulin resistance and DM.[20] In a complementary fashion, exercise training was reported to significantly reduce the risk of developing insulin resistance by improving glucose tolerance and insulin action in individuals at risk for DM.

Prescribed exercise regimens have been advocated for the HIV-1-infected patient, according to stage of disease and current physical health status. Some data have shown that prescribed exercise regimens improve immune measures in HIV-1-infected patients. However, little to no attention to date has been given to the impact of exercise on HIV-1-associated DM risk. One open-label pilot study of 10 men with large abdominal girth used an exercise intervention of progressive resistance training (leg press, leg extension, seated row, and chest press) with an aerobic component three times per week.[21] After 16 weeks of exercise, strength increased for three of the exercises, and there was a significant decrease in total body fat (1.5 kg) – mostly in trunk fat. There were no significant adverse effects. Hence, such interventions may be included within a comprehensive lifestyle management approach to reduce DM risk for the HIV-1-infected patient.

Metabolic syndrome

The metabolic syndrome is a constellation of symptoms previously discussed and has a prevalence in the USA of about 25%. It is characterized by truncal obesity, dyslipidemia, hypertension, and insulin resistance. Increased hepatic lipid output, reduced peripheral lipid uptake, and increased peripheral lipid output all contribute to the dyslipidemia. This cycling of fat generates a metabolic rate about 10% greater than normal. The liver stores the excess fat (associated with hepatic steatosis) and fat is deposited in the muscles (increasing insulin resistance), resulting in a self-perpetuating syndrome.[22] Whereas the etiology remains unknown, it appears to be related to a convergence of metabolic abnormalities occurring with obesity, lack of physical activity, and genetic predisposition. A possible etiology involves parasympathetic/sympathetic tonal balance at the level of the hypothalamus, related to the recent demonstration of a somatotopic organization within the central autonomic nervous system (ANS) such that the intra-abdominal fat pad is innervated by the parasympathetic nervous system and the subcutaneous fat pad is innervated by the sympathetic nervous system.[23] In the general population, the metabolic syndrome has been associated with DM and hypertension risk, CAD, and increased mortality. Essentially, the treatment described for the metabolic syndrome is to treat its components:

- intensify weight management and increase physical activity for the truncal obesity
- treat elevated triglyceride level and/or low HDL cholesterol levels
- treat hypertension
- employ aspirin prophylaxis to reduce the risk for thromboembolism.

Whereas the effects of HIV-1 infection itself and of ARV medications significantly overlap with the symptoms of the metabolic syndrome, HIV-1-associated lipodystrophy syndrome has an independent aspect as well – lipoatrophy. Hence, we will consider the HIV-1-associated lipodystrophy syndrome under HIV-1-specific effects on DM risk below.

Risk factors for diabetes mellitus specific to the HIV-1-infected population

Lipodystrophy syndrome

One of the most recent areas of concern in the field of HIV-1 infection has been the occurrence of glucose intolerance, insulin resistance, and frank DM in response to the current combination ARV medication regimens used to treat HIV-1 infection. Prior to the introduction of CART, long-term health planning seemed irrelevant in HIV/AIDS. Following the introduction of CART, there has been a substantial reduction of the morbidity and mortality due to HIV/AIDS and an increase in the number of individuals surviving into older age (>50 years old).[3] Unfortunately, the price of decreasing morbidity and mortality due to the primary complications of immunosuppression in HIV-1-infected individuals has been the long-term toxicities of these regimens. These toxicities include glucose intolerance, insulin resistance, and DM. Thus, the success of treatment in HIV/AIDS has paradoxically opened the way to a more rapid occurrence of new causes of morbidity and mortality that detracts from the goal of achieving a normal life span for those infected by HIV-1.

In the past 10 years, several types of lipid disorders have been described in persons with HIV-1 infection[24] that are adversely affecting previously established reductions in morbidity and mortality. The dyslipidemia occurring with CART treatment of the HIV-1-infected individual has been variably referred to as the 'lipodystrophy syndrome', the 'metabolic syndrome' and the 'fat redistribution syndrome'. The metabolic abnormalities characteristic of this syndrome include persistently elevated total cholesterol, triglyceride, glucose, C-peptide, and insulin levels and decreased HDL cholesterol levels.[25] Other generally established cardiovascular risk factors – including increased C-reactive protein and homocysteine levels – have also received preliminary study in HIV-1 infection.[26,27] Lipodystrophy syndrome has three subtypes: lipoatrophy syndrome, the syndrome of subcutaneous adiposity, and the mixed syndrome (or fat redistribution syndrome).[28] 'Lipoatrophy syndrome' refers to subcutaneous fat loss (especially in the limbs, face, and buttocks) and deep fat loss visible in the Bichat, preauricular, or orbital fat pads. This deep fat loss may result in pain on mastication, sunken eyeballs, and retro-orbital pain. The syndrome of subcutaneous adiposity occurs without an increase in the visceral adipose tissue (VAT) area and without insulin resistance. It is generally associated with a gain in total body weight less than that observed in classical obesity. The fat redistribution (mixed) syndrome is characterized by a redistribution of fat, with peripheral fat loss (limbs, buttocks, and face, without deep fat loss) and increased VAT. This syndrome has been associated with insulin resistance (similar to that seen in type 2 DM) with elevated insulin, C-peptide, and free fatty acid levels. For our purposes, we shall use the general term C 'lipodystrophy syndrome'.

The prevalence of lipodystrophy syndrome in HIV-1 infection has varied widely, due, in part, to the different methods used in assessing and defining it in research studies. The approach to HIV-1-associated lipodystrophy taken in the Metabolic Change in HIV Infection (FRAM) study by the group of Carl Grunfeld characterized lipoatrophy as an HIV-1-specific phenomenon, separate from central lipohypertrophy.[29] All of the other aspects of the lipodystrophy syndrome are considered consistent with the metabolic syndrome occurring outside of HIV-1 infection. Confirming their approach, dual energy X-ray absorptiometry (DEXA) scanning showed no association between the presence of visceral adiposity (characteristic of the metabolic syndrome) and peripheral lipoatrophy (seen in the HIV-1-infected individuals). More fat was lost in the periphery (legs > arms) so that patients appeared to have a larger trunk (when there may not be increased fat tissue at that site). Peripheral and central lipoatrophy affecting subcutaneous fat was the dominant morphologic change in individuals with HIV-1 infection when compared with individuals without known HIV-1 infection. Progression of HIV-1 infection itself has been associated with the lipodystrophy syndrome. The HIV Outpatient Study showed that of 337 patients with no lipoatrophy at baseline, 13.1% developed moderate or severe lipoatrophy 21 months later. In multivariate analyses, significant risk factors for incident lipoatrophy were white race (OR = 5.2), CD4 cell count 21 months later < 100 cells/mm^3 (OR = 4.2), and BMI < 24 kg/m^2 (OR = 2.4).[30] One hypothesis for the etiology of the disorder is that it results from selective damage by ARV medications to ANS pathways in the CNS innervating either the subcutaneous or visceral fat depots. Greater sympathetic over parasympathetic tone of subcutaneous fat innervation is hypothesized to induce a selective loss of subcutaneous fat (lipoatrophy), and decreased sympathetic over parasympathetic tone of visceral fat innervation induces accumulation of intra-abdominal fat (truncal obesity).[31] However, in the HIV outpatient study, controlling use of or duration of use of any ARV medication (or ARV medication class) as well as clinical HIV-1 disease progression did not affect the results on incident lipoatrophy.[30] Another factor independent of ARV medication use that has been associated with lipoatrophy is tumor necrosis factor gene polymorphisms.

Regarding treatment, the fibrates are as effective in the setting of HIV-1-associated lipodystrophy as they are among those with elevated triglyceride levels without HIV-1 infection. They have a particular indication for isolated and marked hypertriglyceridemia. For elevated LDL cholesterol levels, the statins are indicated at the first line. The issue of drug–drug interactions with the cytochrome P450 3A4 isoenzyme system in the liver and the ARV medications becomes a concern. Pravastatin is the statin least affected by drug interactions and should be the initial statin used,[32] although atorvastatin may be chosen for potency. Simvastatin and lovastatin should not be used with the PIs.[32] Statins also decrease triglyceride levels. Combination therapy of statins and fibrates is used when both LDL cholesterol and triglyceride levels are elevated and when monotherapy fails to achieve target lipid and cholesterol levels. Regarding the potential utility of the insulin sensitizers (the glitazones – rosiglitazone and pioglitazone – and metformin), the results to date have been mixed. Some work suggests that pioglitazone decreases VAT and may be preferable to rosiglitazone. However, further research will be needed to determine what role, if any, these drugs have yet to play.

Antiretroviral medication toxicity

The PIs show an effect on dyslipidemia by drug and by dose. Use of ritonavir as an active PI rather than a booster in a dose of 500 mg orally twice daily is associated with increases of cholesterol of about 25% and of triglycerides of about 200-fold.[22] Nelfinavir is also associated with a dose-dependent increase in triglycerides. However, atazanavir does not appear to be associated with a dyslipidemia, but it has also been associated with asymptomatic hyperbilirubinemia and jaundice. Fosamprenavir, likewise, has been noted to show less of an increase in cholesterol than the other PIs.

Regarding the nRTIs, both stavudine (d4T) and zidovudine (AZT) have been associated with increases in total cholesterol and trigylceride levels, with the greater changes associated with stavudine. In contrast, tenofovir has been shown to decrease total cholesterol levels and increase HDL cholesterol levels.

The non-nucleoside reverse transcriptase inhibitors (NNRTIs) have less concerning effects on fat metabolism than the PIs and the nRTIs. Nevirapine, in fact, given alone, substantially improves the total cholesterol to HDL cholesterol ratio and shows a neutral effect on triglycerides, compared to no effect on the total cholesterol to HDL cholesterol ratio and a modest increase in triglycerides with efavirenz treatment. However, the NNRTIs appear to interact with the PIs so that dyslipidemia is worsened (when using either nevirapine or efavirenz with lopinavir–ritonavir).[22] In addition, a group taking efavirenz and indinavir showed twice the increase in total cholesterol and triglyceride levels as those groups taking either drug alone.

Regarding treatment, if the patient is NNRTI naive, switch to an NNRTI may be indicated and appears to have the greatest positive effects on dyslipidemia of any of the ARV switches that might be chosen. As insulin sensitivity, HDL cholesterol level, and total cholesterol level improve with abacavir, a switch to abacavir in the nRTI backbone might also be considered. If a patient is on a PI and switching within that category is an option, a switch to atazanavir might be indicated.

HCV–HIV-1 co-infection

Another factor exacerbating DM risk appears to be HCV–HIV-1 co-infection, which has become an increasingly frequent clinical concern among HIV-1-infected persons. In addition to its effects on cirrhosis, hepatocellular carcinoma, and mortality, HCV infection also appears to increase the risk of DM (causing an 11-fold increase in those with high risk). In a study of 1230 persons on their first CART regimen, the prevalence of hyperglycemia was significantly higher among HCV–HIV-1 co-infected persons (5.9%) than among HCV-negative persons (3.3%). For participants treated with CART, HCV–HIV-1 co-infection showed an adjusted relative hazard (ARH) of 2.28 for developing hyperglycemia, and PI use showed an independent risk (ARH = 5.02). The incidence of hyperglycemia was highest among HCV–HIV-1 co-infected persons receiving a PI; only one person in this study who was neither HCV–HIV-1 co-infected nor receiving a PI developed hyperglycemia.[33] Another study confirmed this effect with a total of 26 988 veterans.[34] In this study male veterans entering the VA administrative database between 1992 and 2001 were studied. A multivariate Cox regression model showed that the factors associated with DM risk were age (hazards ratio [HR] = 1.44 per 10-year age difference), minority race (HR [Hispanic]; = 1.63, [African American] 1.35), care in the CART era (HR = 2.35), and the interaction of HCV infection and CART era care (HR in the CART era 1.39; in the pre-CART era NS). DM risk might well be expected to be elevated for the HIV-1-infected patient who is older, co-infected with HCV, and prescribed a PI. Hence, HIV-1-infected patients who are HCV co-infected and on PI-containing regimens should be aggressively screened for DM, especially if older.

Complications of diabetes mellitus in HIV-1 infection: implications for clinical management

The long-term consequences of the persistence of the foregoing metabolic abnormalities in patients with HIV-1 infection remain unknown.

There is significant concern that these metabolic abnormalities may represent a significant risk factor for the development not only of CAD and MI but also of other vascular complications, such as CVA.

Coronary artery disease and myocardial infarction

DM has been considered to be a 'CAD equivalent', since the same CAD risk ensues in patients with DM as that reported in patients with prior CAD. HIV-1-infected individuals have multiple sources of CAD risk, as they have an increased frequency of insulin resistance, dyslipidemia, and the metabolic syndrome. A widely cited epidemiologic study in HIV-1 infection, the Multicenter AIDS Cohort Study, reported that HIV-1-infected men on ARV therapy had a two- to three-fold increased risk for hyperglycemia compared with HIV-1-infected individuals not prescribed ARV therapy.[35] A greater than four-fold increase in DM risk compared with HIV-1-seronegative individuals was also noted. Another such study, the Women's Interagency HIV Study, followed 1785 non-pregnant women with no prior history of DM from 1995 to 1998 in four groups:

1. PI users ($n=609$)
2. nRTI-only users ($n=932$)
3. HIV-1-infected women without prior ARV therapy ($n=816$)
4. HIV-1-seronegative women ($n=350$).

The study showed a three-fold increase in incident DM among women on PIs.[36]

Studies on CAD risk are relatively clear in HIV-1-infected individuals; thus, we will turn our focus to MI risk. One study examined the incidence of MI, angina, and CVA in 5672 HIV-1-seropositive patients. Compared with persons not receiving PIs, patients receiving PIs had an increased MI risk (adjusted OR = 4.92), perhaps an increase for angina, but none for CVA.[37] In a study of 73 336 HIV-1-infected French men, exposure to a PI was associated with a higher risk of MI (relative hazard = 2.56). The morbidity ratio relative to the French general male population was 0.8 for PI exposure < 18 months, 1.5 for PI exposure of 18–29 months, and 2.9 for PI exposure ≥ 30 months. With those individuals exposed < 18 months as a reference, the morbidity ratios were 1.9 and 3.6, respectively.[38] Another large study of 4159 HIV-1-infected patients showed that MI rates were not elevated among patients receiving PIs.[39] However, when HIV-1-seropositive and -seronegative patients were compared, the difference in MI rate was higher for HIV-1-seropositive individuals. Hence, this discrepancy could be because risk factors other than use of PIs increase MI risk among HIV-1-seropositive persons, as we have shown for DM risk in this population. It might be considered, then, that the use of the Framingham Heart Study screening tool to monitor 10-year risk for MI and coronary death is warranted on an ongoing basis together with treatment for modifiable DM risk factors in all HIV-1-seropositive patients – not only to prevent DM but also to prevent its clinical sequela of MI.

Cerebrovascular accident

One of the prior studies showed an elevated MI risk without an elevated CVA risk; hence, we now turn our focus to the clinical sequela of CVA in HIV-1-seropositive patients. It is true that an increased incidence of CVA was noted in HIV-1 infection pre-CART. Although uncommon (0.5–7%), CVA was found at a higher-than-expected rate (10–25 per 100 000), controlling for age.[40] However, this research would not have justified any specific preventive management approaches to be taken. In contrast, preventive management of both MI and CVA has taken a prominent focus in the CART era. Despite a number of articles focusing upon MI,[41–44] the long suspected and related possible clinical association with increased CVA risk has only more recently been investigated in HIV-1 infection. An increased prevalence of premature carotid atherosclerosis was found in HIV-1-infected individuals treated with PI-containing regimens for at least 12 months.[45] A pilot study performed by our group confirmed and extended these findings to abnormal cerebral vasomotor reactivity (VMR) using transcranial Doppler sonography (TCD).[46] We compared 21 participants with lipodystrophy syndrome and >18 months of PI exposure to 17 control participants without lipodystrophy syndrome or PI exposure. Participants with lipodystrophy syndrome and PI exposure had statistically significantly more atherosclerotic plaques (68% vs 15%) and greater intima-media thickness (>1 mm; 90% vs 39%) in their common or internal carotid arteries. Regarding TCD results – after adjusting for age, triglyceride level, total cholesterol:HDL cholesterol ratio, C-peptide levels, and the use of lipid-lowering medications – the OR for abnormal VMR remained 1.9 times higher among those with lipodystrophy syndrome and PI exposure than among the control participants.

Although studies of CVA risk factors are available, studies of CVA events in the use of CART regimens remain scant. One cohort study of 772 consecutive HIV-1-infected patients evaluated transient ischemic attack (TIA) and completed CVA rates.[47] A total prevalence of 1.9% (TIA, 0.8%; CVA, 1.2%) was calculated, resulting in an annual incidence rate of 216 per 100 000, with the prevalence highest with advanced clinical HIV-1 disease progression. CVA patients showed worse immunologic status than the TIA patients and the other cohort patients. This study suggested that ischemic CVAs are, indeed, more common in HIV-1-infected patients than in the general population and that this may be partly due to a vasculopathy, which is consistent with an effect related to CART regimen use. The current clinical import of the CVA risk issue in the HIV-1-infected population generally has been described as a 'clockwork bomb that will explode'.[48] This may be expected to be yet more characteristic of the risk for older HIV-1-infected individuals. As with MI risk management, Framingham risk profiles are useful for monitoring purposes in CVA risk management. The recently revised AHA/ASA Stroke Guidelines[49] indicate that each of the components of the metabolic syndrome should be managed, that men should have less than two and women less than one alcoholic beverage daily, that snoring should be monitored (as sleep apnea associated with obesity is a CVA risk factor), that weight should be controlled, and that 75 mg of aspirin daily be used to treat a 5-year CVA risk of >3% or a 10-year CVA risk of >10%. Further research in this important area is warranted.

Psychiatric implications and treatments

Studies of the comorbidity of DM with psychopathology show that psychiatric patients with mood disorders, particularly depressive disorders, were more likely to suffer from DM and cardiovascular illness than those diagnosed with schizophrenia or psychiatric disorders due to a medical condition.[50] The frequency of DM in hospitalized patients diagnosed with bipolar affective disorder is also higher than in the general population. One study focused on bipolar affective disorder and demonstrated that patients with comorbid DM had significantly more lifetime psychiatric hospitalizations than non-diabetic patients.[51] Bipolar disorder patients with DM had a more severe course. The cause of this overlapping comorbidity in the general population remains a source of speculation at the present time.

Comorbidity of diabetes mellitus with psychiatric disorders in HIV-1 infection

The relationship of DM to depressive disorders may have an underlying pathophysiologic basis. Major depressive disorder is known to be associated with hypercortisolemia, which, in turn, is associated with elevated glucose levels. One recent study supported the hypothesis that hypercortisolemia is associated with an increased DM risk in patients with depressive disorders.[52] It showed that glucose concentration was positively associated with mean morning cortisol concentrations and negatively associated with a measure of insulin receptor sensitivity. Whereas it should be cautioned that stimulatory influences on the limbic–hypothalamic–pituitary–adrenal (LHPA) axis are complex and that negative feedback regulation by glucocorticoids is diverse, the relationship between major depressive disorder (at least), cortisol level, and DM risk could be mediated though this axis. Both the hypothalamus and, secondarily, the hippocampus are involved in regulation of the LHPA axis. HIV-1 infection is independently associated with higher neuronal destruction associated with higher levels of CD4 receptor in the hippocampus, which is also susceptible to neuronal cell death due to aging effects and due to the neurotoxic effects of chronically high levels of glucocorticoids associated with major depressive disorder.[53,54] High levels of life stressors are also known to be associated with chronically elevated glucocorticoid levels in addition to major depressive disorder. Thus, a constellation of predisposing factors involving high life stressor burden, major depressive disorder, older age, and HIV-1 infection may be interacting with one another to produce a diathesis to chronically elevated glucose levels and high DM risk.

Psychiatric interventions to reduce depression and weight in HIV-1 infection

A number of psychotropic medications are associated with weight gain, particularly the tricylic antidepressants (TCAs), certain mood-stabilizing medications, and the atypical antipsychotic medications (see next section). Weight gain has been noted to occur throughout the TCA class, although the secondary amine TCAs (such as desipramine and nortriptyline) show less weight gain than the tertiary amine TCAs (such as imipramine and amitriptyline). Regarding the mood-stabilizing agents, weight gain is a significant concern with lithium and valproate as well as (though to a lesser extent) with carbamazepine. Regarding antidepressant treatments of choice in HIV-1-seropositive individuals with DM, catecholamines increase glucose, reduce insulin release, and reduce insulin sensitivity. In contrast, higher serotonergic transmission is associated with decreased plasma glucose levels and increased insulin sensitivity. This suggests the expected utility of the selective serotonin reuptake inhibitors (SSRIs); however, it should be noted that non-depressed obese patients treated with SSRIs other than fluoxetine showed no significant weight reduction effects and that studies of SSRIs for food craving have been similarly disappointing.[55] Six studies of fluoxetine at a dose of 60 mg/day demonstrated weight reduction (up to 9.3 kg), fasting plasma glucose level reduction (upto 45 mg%), and HbA_{1c} reduction (upto 2.5%).[56] These results have been shown to extend to other SSRIs, such as sertraline and paroxetine. In addition, the SSRIs do not pose a significant concern for hypertension as a factor complicating or exacerbating DM (outside of the acute, severe toxicity associated with serotonin syndrome). Likewise, the SSRIs are not expected to cause or exacerbate a tendency toward DM risk due to physical inactivity, as they are associated with nervousness and restlessness (rather than with the sedation commonly noted with the TCAs). A placebo-controlled trial of paroxetine in diabetic patients showed a trend toward greater control of glucose level, higher levels of sex hormone binding globulin (indicative of higher insulin sensitivity), and, interestingly, a trend toward lower serum cortisol levels.[57] Given that paroxetine is also less likely to have drug–drug interactions with the ARV medications than most other antidepressants, it may be the antidepressant of choice for HIV-1-seropositive patients with DM, although sertraline might also be advocated.

The setting of treating the HIV-1-seropositive DM patient might well also be complicated by the presence of painful peripheral neuropathy. The latter may be due to HIV-1 infection itself, and/or to treatment with the dideoxynucleoside ARV medications (stavudine, didanosine, and zalcitabine) as well as to the lipodystrophy syndrome associated with DM due to the PIs, and/or pre-existing DM. The choice of antidepressants in the setting of painful peripheral neuropathy would generally be those that enhance both noradrenergic and serotonergic transmission. However, enhanced noradrenergic transmission is suboptimal for glucose management. Hence, it might be recommended that treatment of neuropathic pain in HIV-1 infection be focused more specifically upon serotenergic transmission together with the use of other medication classes, such as the anticonvulsants. In particular, lamotrigine has been reported to be effective in several forms of neuropathic pain, including diabetic neuropathy, post-CVA pain, and trigeminal neuralgia. In a double-blind, placebo-controlled trial of painful HIV-1-associated distal sensory polyneuropathy, lamotrigine was also shown to be both effective and well tolerated.[58] Thus, lamotrigine may be added to paroxetine (or sertraline) when treating the HIV-1-seropositive patient with DM, depressive disorder, and painful peripheral neuropathy.

It should also be noted that older age has been independently associated with clinically apparent (i.e. symptomatic) DSP in HIV-1-infected individuals. Of further clinical relevance, peripheral neuropathy has been demonstrated to be a true risk factor for falls in the elderly. Moreover, the pain associated with DSP has been reported to be a significant cause of decreased adherence to CART regimens as well. Thus, the tetrad of older age, DM, depressive disorder, and painful peripheral neuropathy may prove yet more clinically important to manage. It may be noted that paroxetine and sertraline as well as lamotrigine can be used with safety in treating older patients, when appropriate dosage adjustments are made upon treatment initiation and escalation (as indicated by individualized treatment response).

Atypical antipsychotics and diabetes mellitus risk in HIV-1 infection

Use of antipsychotic medications is of importance to consider as well as the antidepressants among the HIV-1-infected patient population. Antipsychotic medications are used for the treatment of bipolar affective disorder (associated with an increased DM risk), psychotic symptoms associated with severe HIV-1-associated dementia, chronic pain associated with peripheral neuropathy (or other painful HIV-1-associated conditions), and the persistent psychotic symptoms of the severely mentally ill (who are at increased risk for HIV-1 infection due to a relative lack of use of HIV risk behavior precautions). The conventional antipsychotic medications are generally avoided in HIV-1-infected individuals due to the high degree of neuroleptic sensitivity displayed by these patients to extrapyramidal symptoms, which is related to the damage caused by HIV-1 infection in the basal ganglia. However, the atypical antipsychotic medications present an alternative toxicity issue to be considered as well – that of glucose intolerance and an increased risk for developing (or exacerbating existing) DM. Clozapine and olanzapine are particularly liable to this side effect. In fact, clozapine has been associated with the development of diabetic ketoacidosis, which was reversed with drug discontinuation and recurred with reinstitution of drug. In contrast, DM risk is only moderately high for quetiapine and rather low for risperidone although it is lowest for ziprasidone and aripiprazole.[59] Regarding extrapyramidal symptoms, outside of risperidone, the atypical neuroleptics as a class are largely free of extrapyramidal reactions (except at the high end of the dosing range). Ziprasidone may be preferred, if use of the intramuscular route is a potential to consider. Interestingly, studies to date among older patients at yet higher DM risk have not documented the increased DM risk of the atypical antipsychotics, compared to that seen in younger samples.[60] This may be due to the impact of aging being greater than the impact of the metabolic side effects of the atypical neuroleptics.[55] The foregoing atypical antipsychotic use recommendations for HIV-1-infected individuals with DM differ from those made for the elderly patient population generally, where experts prefer risperidone, with quetiapine high on the second line.[61] For the newly developing setting of older HIV-1-infected individuals with DM requiring long-term management, we would maintain the recommendation for ziprasidone or aripiprazole made for their younger counterparts. For the subgroup of older HIV-1-infected patients with DM and QTc prolongation or congestive heart failure, aripiprazole may be preferred.[62]

Summary

The three-way intersection of HIV-1 infection, DM, and psychiatric disorders has become increasingly common in the CART era. We have considered the issue from the point of view of examining the treatment of risk factors for DM that might be expected to ameliorate the clinical impact on HIV-1-infected persons, generally, as well as those with psychiatric disorders, specifically. Whereas little can be done regarding the non-modifiable DM risk factors of age, ethnicity, family history, and other clinical conditions associated with insulin resistance (acanthosis nigricans and polycystic ovary syndrome), a great impact can be made upon the modifiable DM risk factors. Total body weight (and fat), exercise level, and cigarette smoking are important lifestyle factors for which the management chosen has verifiable effects on DM risk. Although gestational diabetes could be reduced by avoidance of pregnancy, ethically and morally, the support of the choice to carry through a pregnancy in the CART era is well justified. The management of lipid levels and hypertension, particularly in the setting of the metabolic syndrome, is also of notable import in reducing DM risk. There are three contributors to HIV-1-specific DM risk. The counterpart of the metabolic syndrome for DM risk among HIV-1-seronegative individuals is lipodystrophy syndrome in HIV-1-seropositive individuals, with the only differentiating factor being the addition of lipoatrophy among HIV-1-seropositive persons. In addition, and associated with the occurrence of lipodystrophy syndrome, is ARV medication toxicity. Finally, HCV–HIV-1 co-infection must be considered in managing DM risk among HIV-1-seropositive persons. Gemfibrozil should be used to manage elevated triglyceride levels and the statins should be used to manage the total cholesterol : HDL cholesterol ratio (with caution for the statins regarding drug–drug interactions with the ARV medications).

The intersection with the psychiatric disorders revolves around the depressive disorders, bipolar affective disorder, HIV-1-associated dementia with psychotic symptoms, and severe, persistent, pre-existing psychotic disorders. For depressive disorders, the SSRIs offer an advantage in DM risk management, particularly paroxetine and sertraline. Lamotrigine may be added for chronic pain from peripheral neuropathy associated with HIV-1 infection itself, ARV medication toxicity (dideoxynucleoside nRTIs and PI-associated lipodystrophy syndrome with DM), and/or pre-existing DM. For disorders in which antipsychotics are of proven utility, ziprasidone (which has an intramuscular route available) and aripiprazole may be the drugs of choice. Older age is more common now than ever before among HIV-1-infected individuals and is an independent risk factor for DM, CAD, MI, CVA, and peripheral neuropathy (with associated falls). Pharmacologic management requires greater caution in this rapidly growing subpopulation of HIV-1-infected individuals. Regarding atypical antipsychotic choice, ziprasidone and aripiprazole remain favored.

This work was supported by NIH grants MH58532 and MH/AG 61629.

References

1. Centers for Disease Control and Prevention: HIV/AIDS Surveillance Report, 2004. Atlanta: US Department of Health and Human Services, Centers for Disease Control and Prevention; 2005; 16: 1–46.
2. Miami-Dade County Health Dept. HIV/AIDS Surveillance Report. http://www.dadehealth.org/downloads/MAR-06.pdf, 2006. accessed March 2006.
3. Goodkin K, Wilkie FL, Concha M et al. Aging and neuro-AIDS conditions: a potential interaction with the changing spectrum of HIV-1 associated morbidity and mortality in the era of HAART? J Clin Epidemiol 2001; 54: S35–43.
4. Lavery LA, van Houtum WH, Ashry HR et al. Diabetes-related lower-extremity amputations disproportionately affect Blacks and Mexican Americans. South Med J 1999; 92(6): 593–9.
5. Schraer CD, Risica PM, Ebbesson SO et al. Low fasting insulin levels in Eskimos compared to American Indians: are Eskimos less insulin resistant? Int J Circumpolar Health 1999; 58(4): 272–80.
6. Hariri S, Yoon PW, Qureshi N et al. Family history of type 2 diabetes: a population-based screening tool for prevention? Genet Med 2006; 8(2): 102–8.
7. Stuart CA, Driscoll MS, Lundquist KF et al. Acanthosis nigricans. J Basic Clin Physiol Pharmacol 1998; 9(2–4): 407–18.
8. Charnvises K, Weerakiet S, Tingthanatikul Y et al. Acanthosis nigricans: clinical predictor of abnormal glucose tolerance in Asian women with polycystic ovary syndrome. Gyn Endocrinol 2005; 21(3): 161–4.
9. Hu FB, Manson JE, Stampfer MJ et al. Diet lifestyle and the risk of type II diabetes in women. N Engl J Med 2001; 345: 790–7.
10. Weinstein AR, Sesso HD, Lee IM et al. Relationship of physical activity vs body mass index with type 2 diabetes in women. JAMA 2004; 292: 1188–94.
11. Devroey D, De Swaef N, Coigniez P et al. Correlations between lipid levels and age, gender, glycemia, obesity, diabetes, and smoking. Endocrine Res 2004; 30(1): 83–93.
12. Lyerly AD, Anderson J. Human immunodeficiency virus and assisted reproduction: reconsidering evidence, reframing ethics. Fertil Steril 2001; 75(5): 843–58.
13. Garcia-Puig J, Ruilope LM, Luque M et al. AVANT Study Group Investigators. Glucose metabolism in patients with essential hypertension. Am J Med 2006; 119(4): 318–26.
14. Tirosh A, Shai I, Tekes-Manova D et al. Israeli Diabetes Research Group. Normal fasting plasma glucose levels and type 2 diabetes in young men. N Engl J Med 2005; 353(14): 1454–62.

15. Perry IJ, Wannamethee SG, Walker MK et al. Prospective study of risk factors for development of non-insulin dependent diabetes in middle aged British men. BMJ 1995; 310(6979): 560–4.

16. Cicero AF, Dormi A, Nascetti S et al. Relative role of major risk factors for Type 2 diabetes development in the historical cohort of the Brisighella Heart Study: an 8-year follow-up. Diabet Med 2005; 22(9): 1263–6.

17. Grunfeld C, Kotler DP, Shigenaga JK et al. Circulating interferon-alpha levels and hypertriglyceridemia in the acquired immunodeficiency syndrome. Am J Med 1991; 90(2): 154–62.

18. Patja K, Jousilahti P, Hu G et al. Effects of smoking, obesity and physical activity on the risk of type 2 diabetes in middle-aged Finnish men and women. J Int Med 2005; 258(4): 356–62.

19. Niaura R, Shadel WG, Morrow K et al. Human immunodeficiency virus infection, AIDS, and smoking cessation: the time is now. Clin Infect Dis 2000; 31(3): 808–12.

20. Hawley JA. Exercise as a therapeutic intervention for the prevention and treatment of insulin resistance. Diabetes Metab Res Rev 2004; 20(5): 383–93.

21. Roubenoff R, Weiss L, McDermott A et al. A pilot study of exercise training to reduce trunk fat in adults with HIV-associated fat redistribution. AIDS 1999; 13(11): 1373–5.

22. Moyle G. A review of the aetiology of dyslipidaemia and hyperlipidaemia in patients with HIV. Int J STD AIDS 2005; 16(Suppl 1): 14–22.

23. Kreier F, Fliers E, Voshol PJ et al. Selective parasympathetic innervation of subcutaneous and intra-abdominal fat – functional implications. J Clin Invest 2002; 110(9): 1243–50.

24. Carr A, Samaras K, Chisholm DJ et al. Pathogenesis of HIV-1-protease inhibitor-associated peripheral lipodystrophy, hyperlipidaemia, and insulin resistance. Lancet 1998; 352: 1881–3.

25. Carr A, Samaras K, Thorisdottir A et al. Diagnosis, prediction, and natural course of HIV-1 protease-inhibitor-associated lipodystrophy, hyperlipidaemia, and diabetes mellitus: a cohort study. Lancet 1999; 353: 2093–9.

26. Vigouroux C, Gharakhanian S, Salhi Y et al. Diabetes, insulin resistance and dyslipidaemia in lipodystrophic HIV-infected patients on highly active antiretroviral therapy (HAART). Diabetes Metab 1999; 25(3): 225–32.

27. Mercie P, Thiebaut R, Lavignolle V et al. Evaluation of cardiovascular risk factors in HIV-1 infected patients using carotid intima-media thickness measurement. Ann Med 2002; 34(1): 55–63.

28. Saint-Marc T, Partisani M, Poizot-Martin I et al. Fat distribution evaluated by computed tomography and metabolic abnormalities in patients undergoing antiretroviral therapy: preliminary results of the LIPOCO study. AIDS 2000; 14(1): 37–49.

29. Tien PC, Grunfeld C. What is HIV-associated lipodystrophy? Defining fat redistribution changes in HIV infection. Curr Opin Infect Dis 2004; 17: 27–32.

30. Lichtenstein KA, Delaney KM, Armon C et al. Incidence of and risk factors for lipoatrophy (abnormal fat loss) in ambulatory HIV-1-infected patients. J Acquir Immune Defic Syndr 2003; 32(1): 48–56.

31. Fliers E, Sauerwein HP, Romijn JA et al. HIV-associated adipose redistribution syndrome as a selective autonomic neuropathy. Lancet 2003; 362(9397): 1758–60.

32. Wlodarczyk D. Managing medical conditions associated with Cardiac Risk in Patients with HIV. HIV InSite Knowledge Base Chapter. UCSF Center for HIV Information: August 2004. http://hivinsite.ucsf.edu/InSite.

33. Mehta SH, Moore RD, Thomas DL et al. The effect of HAART and HCV infection on the development of hyperglycemia among HIV-infected persons. J Acquir Immune Defic Syndr 2003; 33(5): 577–84.
34. Butt AA, Fultz SL, Kwoh CK et al. Risk of diabetes in HIV infected veterans pre- and post-HAART and the role of HCV coinfection. Hepatology 2004; 40(1): 115–19.
35. Brown TT, Cole SR, Li X et al. Antiretroviral therapy and the prevalence and incidence of diabetes mellitus in the multicenter AIDS cohort study. Arch Int Med 2005; 165(10): 1179–84.
36. Justman JE, Benning L, Danoff A et al. Protease inhibitor use and the incidence of diabetes mellitus in a large cohort of HIV-infected women. J Acquir Immune Defic Syndr 2003; 32: 298–302.
37. Holmberg SD, Moorman AC, Williamson JM et al. Protease inhibitors and cardiovascular outcomes in patients with HIV-1. Lancet 2002; 360: 1747–8.
38. Mary-Krause M, Cotte L, Simon A et al. Increased risk of myocardial infarction with duration of protease inhibitor therapy in HIV-infected men. AIDS 2003; 17(17): 2479–86.
39. Klein D, Hurley LB, Quesenberry CP et al. Do protease inhibitors increase the risk for coronary heart disease in patients with HIV-1 infection? J Acquir Immune Defic Syndr 2002; 30: 471–7.
40. Berger JR, Harris JO, Gregorios J et al. Cerebrovascular disease in AIDS: a case control study. AIDS 1990; 4: 239–44.
41. Henry K, Melroe H, Huebusch J et al. Severe premature coronary artery disease with protease inhibitors. Lancet 1998; 351: 1328.
42. Passalaris JD, Sepkowitz KA, Glesby MJ. Coronary artery disease and human immunodeficiency virus infection. Clin Infec Dis 2000; 31: 787–97.
43. Behrens G, Schmidt H, Meyer D et al. Vascular complications associated with the use of HIV protease inhibitors. Lancet 1998; 351: 1958.
44. Duong M, Buisson M, Cottin Y et al. Coronary heart disease associated with the use of human immunodeficiency virus (HIV)-1 protease inhibitors: report of four cases and review. Clin Cardiol 2001; 24(10): 690–4.
45. Maggi P, Serio G, Epifani G et al. Premature lesions of the carotid vessels in HIV-1-infected patients treated with protease inhibitors. AIDS 2000; 14(16): F123–8.
46. Concha M, Symes S, Goodkin K et al. Risk of cerebrovascular disease in HIV-1-infected subjects with lipodystrophy syndrome and long-term exposure to protease inhibitors (P213). Stroke 2003; 34(1): 295.
47. Evers S, Nabavi D, Rahmann A et al. Ischemic cerebrovascular events in HIV infection. Cerebrovasc Dis 2003; 15: 99–205.
48. Maggi P, Fiorentino G, Epifani G et al. Premature vascular lesions in HIV-positive patients: a clockwork bomb that will explode? AIDS 2002; 16(6): 947–8.
49. Sacco RL, Adams R, Albers G et al. AHA/ASA Guidelines. Guidelines for prevention of stroke in patients with ischemic stroke or transient ischemic attack: a statement for healthcare professionals from the American Heart Association/American Stroke Association Council on Stroke. Stroke 2006; 37: 577–617.
50. Adamis D, Ball C. Physical morbidity in elderly psychiatric inpatients: prevalence and possible relations between the major mental disorders and physical illness. Int J Geriatric Psychiatry 2000; 15(3): 248–53.
51. Cassidy F, Ahearn E, Carroll BJ. Elevated frequency of diabetes mellitus in hospitalized manic-depressive patients. Am J Psychiatry 1999; 156(9): 1417–20.

52. Weber-Hamann B, Kopf D, Lederbogen F et al. Activity of the hypothalamus–pituitary–adrenal system and oral glucose tolerance in depressed patients. Neuroendocrinology 2005; 81(3): 200–4.
53. Goodkin K, Antoni MH, Helder L et al. Psychoneuroimmunological aspects of disease progression among women with human papillomavirus-associated cervical dysplasia and human immunodeficiency virus type 1 co-infection. Int J Psychiatry Med 1993; 23(2): 119–48.
54. Goodkin K, Shapshak P, Fujimura RK et al. Immune function, brain, and HIV-1 infection. In: Goodkin K, Visser A (eds.) Psychoneuroimmunology: Stress, Mental Disorders and Health. Washington, DC: American Psychiatric Press, 2000; 243–316.
55. Zimmermann U, Kraus T, Himmerich H et al. Epidemiology, implications and mechanisms underlying drug-induced weight gain in psychiatric patients. J Psychiatric Res 2003; 37(3): 193–220.
56. Goodnick PJ. Use of antidepressants in treatment of comorbid diabetes mellitus and depression as well as in diabetic neuropathy. Ann Clin Psychiatry 2001; 13(1): 31–41.
57. Paile-Hyvarinen M, Wahlbeck K, Eriksson JG. Quality of life and metabolic status in mildly depressed women with type 2 diabetes treated with paroxetine: a single-blind randomised placebo controlled trial. BMC Fam Pract 2003; 4: 7.
58. Simpson DM, McArthur JC, Olney R et al. Lamotrigine for HIV-associated painful sensory neuropathies: a placebo-controlled trial. Neurology 2003; 60(9): 1508–14.
59. Simpson GM. Atypical antipsychotics and the burden of disease. Am J Manag Care 2005; 11(8 Suppl): S235–41.
60. Micca JL, Hoffmann VP, Lipkovich I et al. Retrospective analysis of diabetes risk in elderly patients with dementia in olanzapine clinical trials. Am J Geriatr Psychiatry 2006; 14(1): 62–70.
61. Alexopoulos GS, Streim J, Carpenter D et al. Using antipsychotic agents in older patients. J Clin Psychiatry 2004; 65(Suppl 2): 5–99.
62. Travis MJ, Burns T, Dursun S et al. Aripiprazole in schizophrenia: consensus guidelines. Int J Clin Practice 2005; 59(4): 485–95.

Chapter 8

Nutritional interventions for individuals with mental illness and diabetes mellitus

Louise P Grant

Psychiatric disorders and diabetes mellitus: challenges for nutritional interventions

In the USA approximately 20.8 million persons are estimated to have diabetes mellitus (DM). Nearly one-third are undiagnosed. The total combined direct and indirect costs associated with DM approximates $132 billion annually.[1] An increased prevalence of DM has been observed in patients also diagnosed with mental illness. Major depressive disorders have been observed in 10–15% of those diagnosed with DM, which is about twice the rate found in the general population.[2] Anxiety, other mood disorders, and dementia are associated with an increased risk for diabetes.[3,4] Schizophrenia, in particular, has been associated with insulin resistance and glucose intolerance, with a tendency towards developing DM.[4,5] There are several nutritional reasons for this increased association between psychiatric disorders and DM.

Patients with psychiatric disorders exhibit overall higher rates of obesity, poorer quality of dietary intake, and lower levels of physical activity, as well as greater smoking behavior than the general adult population, thus increasing the overall risk of diabetes. Many medications used to treat psychiatric disorders are associated with development of weight gain, glucose intolerance, and diabetes. Atypical antipsychotics have been particularly implicated in weight gain and treatment-emergent DM.[6] The fear of weight gain associated with medications may limit patient adherence to medication management for mental illness. As the symptoms of mental illness worsen, the patient is less adherent to medical management of diabetes, with poorer diabetes outcomes.[7] Furthermore, it has been observed that patients with co-occurring mental illness are less likely to receive evidence-based, recommended diabetes-related interventions.[8]

For example, major depression was associated with less physical activity, poorer dietary choices, and lower adherence to oral hypo-glycemia, antihypertensive, and lipid-lowering medications. Severity of depression appears to be directly related to poorer adherence to dietary recommendations as measured by number of days of non-adherence to oral hypoglycemic regimens, poorer physical and mental functioning, and higher health care costs.[9] There is a higher failure in weight management programs in patients with both depression and type 2 DM than in those without depression.[10]

Clinical findings in a patient with DM that suggest that there may be an underlying or unrecognized psychiatric illness include:

- persistent elevations of hemoglobin A_{1c} (HbA_{1c})
- erratic fluctuations in blood glucose
- persistent weight gain
- dietary recommendation non-adherence
- frequent diabetic crisis episodes
- repeated failure to carry out recommended clinical testing.

An additional barrier to DM management among the mentally ill is the high degree of associated homelessness. Homeless persons with DM exhibit poorer glycemic control, often related to the type of food served in shelters and the inability to be selective about dietary choices. Additionally, the scheduling and logistics of insulin use, obtaining and keeping diabetic supplies, and the inability to coordinate insulin and hypoglycemic medication intake with meals[11] contribute significantly to poorer DM outcomes.

Careful disease self-management of DM can reduce the complications of DM that contribute to morbidity, disability, and mortality,[4] even among patients with mental illness. A health care provider working with this population, however, must recognize and be willing to address the unique challenges in DM self-management experienced by patients with mental illness. These include treatment adherence barriers, personal neglect, personal and systemic barriers to health care access, confusion regarding care instructions, and psychosocial complexities that undermine effective care of DM. Lack of control of either DM or mental illness exacerbates or complicates one or the other, and, frequently, both. For this reason, a team-based, coordinated care, case management approach, located in a single site is highly recommended and effective.[4] This chapter will focus on the basics of medical nutrition therapy for patients with co-occurring mental illness and DM with an emphasis on practical applications for the healthcare team.

Medical nutrition therapy for diabetes mellitus

Medical nutrition therapy (MNT) services are defined as 'nutritional diagnostic, therapy, and counseling services for the purpose of disease management which are furnished by a registered dietitian or nutrition professional.'[12] The primary focus of MNT for DM is on the effort the individual makes to adopt healthy eating habits that lead to improved DM control, lower serum lipids, and achieving blood pressure goals. Effective MNT for DM utilizes American Dietetic Association (ADA) Nutrition Practice Guidelines and incorporates these five primary clinical goals:

1. achieve and maintain near-normal blood glucose
2. achieve optimal serum lipid levels
3. provide adequate caloric intake
4. prevent, delay, or treat nutrition-related diabetes complications
5. improve or maintain overall health through optimal nutrition.

Implementation of these guidelines has been shown to result in a 1–2% decrease in HbA_{1c} levels (resulting in levels of 7–8%). This is similar to the outcomes seen with oral hypoglycemic medications. In addition, moderate reductions in dietary sodium intake (2400 mg/day) can lead to significant decreases in blood pressure. This is particularly important for individuals who are 'salt sensitive', a frequently found characteristic of many persons with diabetes.

As with any diabetes regimen, nutrition recommendations must be tailored to the needs of the individual. The nutrition intervention typically consists of an average of three counseling sessions with a registered dietitian, over 3–6 months. At the initial visit, the registered dietitian conducts a thorough assessment of the person's educational level, individual circumstances, personal, cultural, and ethnic preferences and lifestyle, usual food intake, metabolic and personal goals, and, importantly, the willingness to change to achieve the goals of MNT.[4,13] A discussion then follows to identify the barriers encountered by the individual with diabetes in making healthy food choices, and the ways in which these eating habits can realistically be modified. The dietitian attempts to work with the patient to jointly solve nutrition-related problems, identify the patient's specific goals, and then develop a balanced meal plan. As with other diabetes treatments, the effectiveness of the meal plan is assessed using serum glucose and lipid levels, and blood pressure. The impact of MNT on improved metabolic control is usually seen 6–12 weeks after the initial visit. Annual sessions may be needed to reinforce the goals. Persons with mental illness may require an increased number or frequency of sessions with the registered dietitian.

Type 1 diabetes mellitus

For patients with type 1 DM, there is an emphasis on integrating the insulin regimen into the client's lifestyle. The total carbohydrate content of the meals (and snacks) is the major determinant of insulin requirements. Once the amount of insulin required to cover the patient's usual meal carbohydrate is determined, the patient can be taught how to vary premeal rapid-acting insulin doses, based on the planned carbohydrate content of the meal (these are the so-called insulin-to-carbohydrate ratios). This type of management is associated with positive effects on quality of life and psychological well-being, despite an increased number of injections and blood glucose monitoring. For persons receiving a fixed insulin regimen, consistency of carbohydrate intake is highly recommended. Fixed insulin regimens are preferred for patients with mental illness, due to the increased consistency, ease of administration, and greater level of structure, particularly for patients where homelessness is an issue.

Type 2 diabetes mellitus

For patients with type 2 DM, the emphasis is on lifestyle changes that will enhance diabetes control. MNT with this population begins with strategies that reduce caloric intake, and increase energy expenditure through physical activity. Weight loss, particularly intra-abdominal fat, reduces insulin resistance and improves dyslipidemias in short-term studies. Long-term data, however, are lacking. Recent data from the Diabetes Prevention Program demonstrated that low-fat diets, increased physical activity, ongoing educational sessions, and frequent participant contact were needed to sustain a 5–7% weight loss over 2–3 years.[14] In working with patients who have mental illness and diabetes, MNT is usually implemented by a registered dietitian who is a part of the health care team. It is also highly recommended, however, that the entire health care team have knowledge of MNT,[4,13] so that all members of the health care team can reinforce the clinical goals at each patient contact.

Benefits of diabetes mellitus medical nutrition therapy

Patients receiving MNT according to nutrition care practice guidelines consistently demonstrate significant improvements in fasting plasma glucose (FPG) control, HbA_{1c} levels, and significant improvements in cholesterol values.[15] This is particularly evident when the intervention includes increased time and/or the number of sessions with a registered dietitian who provides diabetes-related medical nutrition therapy.[16] Achieving the clinical goals of MNT leads to the prevention of the chronic complications of DM, including obesity, hypertension, dyslipidemias, cardiovascular disease, and nephropathy. Additional outcomes include improved perceived self-health status and fewer missed workdays at 6-month evaluations. In 2002, in the USA, the Federal government determined that the benefits derived from MNT were sufficient to warrant coverage under Medicare Part B for patients diagnosed with type 1, type 2, or gestational diabetes (defined in diagnostic criteria for diabetes as a fasting glucose = 126 mg/dl).[12]

Recommendations regarding dietary composition and planning

A meta-analysis of recommendations regarding diet, particularly carbohydrate and fiber content, indicated that blood glucose, lipid levels, and HbA_{1c} levels improved best when a high-fiber, high-carbohydrate diet was followed.[17] More than half the calories in the diet should be from carbohydrate sources. Protein should constitute about 15% and

Table 8.1 Recommended distribution and sources of dietary energy (calories) and fiber

Nutrient	Calories (% of total energy intake)	Food sources
Carbohydrate	55–65%	Whole grains and breads, fresh fruits, vegetables, low-fat milk (2%, 1% or skim milk)
Protein[a]	11–18%	Meats, poultry, fish, dairy products, eggs, legumes, soy-based foods
Fats[b] – divided equally between:	25–30%	
Saturated fats		Beef, pork, veal, poultry, butter, dairy products, coconut, palm and palm kernel oil
Unsaturated fats		Olives, olive oil, canola oil
Polyunsaturated fats		Nuts, seeds, vegetable oils, i.e. soybean, safflower, corn, flax and fish oils
Dietary fiber	25–50 g/day	Oats, barley, whole-grain breads, cereals, pastas, brown rice, dry beans, peas, lentils, nuts, fruits, vegetables

[a]In presence of diabetic nephropathy, protein should not exceed 0.8 g/kg, or 10% total kcal.
[b]Less than 10% of energy should come from saturated fats. If low-density lipoprotein (LDL) cholesterol ≥ 100 g/dl, adjust saturated fat level to < 7% energy.

fat sources should account for no more than 25–30% of total energy intake (Table 8.1). Whenever possible, patients should be encouraged to limit alcohol intake to one 'standard drink' (12 oz of beer, 5 oz of wine, 1.5 oz of 80 proof spirits) for women and no more than two standard drinks per day for men. For individuals who take insulin or insulin secretagogues, alcohol should be consumed with food to prevent hypoglycemia. Evening consumption of alcohol can also increase the risk of hypoglycemia the next morning, so that blood glucose testing at this time should be to determine if a reduction in the morning insulin dose might be needed.

In recent years increasing attention has been given to the increase in *trans* fatty acids in the average diet in industrialized societies. *Trans* fatty acids are unsaturated fatty acids formed when vegetable oils are processed and hydrogenated. Evidence suggests that increasing ratios of these *trans* fatty acids tend to adversely affect total cholesterol concentrations and low-density lipoprotein : high density lipoprotein (LDL : HDL) cholesterol ratios.[18] As a result, it is prudent to recommend to patients that they minimize intake of foods that contain hydrogenated fats/*trans* fatty acids, such as traditional stick margarine and vegetable shortenings that have been subjected to hydrogenation. Foods that are major contributors of hydrogenated *trans* fatty acids in the diet include pastries and fried foods such as doughnuts and French fries, whole milk, whole milk cheeses, butter, and meats. Patients who eat one or more daily meals from fast food restaurants are likely to have diets high in fats, particularly those containing *trans* fatty acids. Additionally, patients should be encouraged to restrict dietary cholesterol intake to < 300 mg/day. If LDL cholesterol levels are > 100 g/dl, then dietary cholesterol should be < 200 mg/day.

ADA evidence-based practice guidelines strongly recommend accommodating the life stage of the patient in planning and implementing dietary changes.[19] This is particularly true for adolescents with type 2 DM, who should be encouraged to change eating and physical activity habits that decrease insulin resistance and improve metabolic status. For the diabetic adolescent with co-occurring psychiatric illness, the maintenance of a healthy weight, while also encouraging normal growth and development, is particularly challenging to the health care team. Careful integrated coordination is needed to ensure a reasonable level of adherence to medications required to address DM and mental illness, as well as special attention to diet and physical activity.

For older adults, therapy should provide for nutritional and psychological needs. For patients at risk for type 2 DM, MNT should decrease this risk by encouraging physical activity and by promoting food choices that will facilitate moderate weight loss and/or prevent weight gain. Individuals treated with insulin or insulin secretagogues should be provided frequent self-management education to treat and prevent hypoglycemia, acute illness, and exercise-related blood glucose problems. Overall, it is the total amount of carbohydrate in the diet that is more important than the type. This is a departure from past recommendations and can result in some resistance from long-term diabetic patients accustomed to restricting certain types of carbohydrates. It is best to operate within the patient's frame of reference and assess the patient's readiness to change prior to introducing new (to the patient) concepts of carbohydrate intake management. Evaluations of successful nutrition education interventions for older adults have revealed that positive outcomes were more likely when nutrition messages were limited, simple, practical, and directed to the specific needs of the participants. Individuals who appeared to be more motivated at the outset appeared more likely to be successful in achieving dietary changes.[20]

The importance of controlling weight must be emphasized. Maintaining a body mass index (BMI) ≤ 25 is recommended; BMI = weight (kg)/height (m^2). Modest weight loss, even a loss of just 10 lb (4.5 kg), has been shown to be effective in reducing blood glucose levels and insulin resistance. Studies have consistently demonstrated that patients with schizophrenia do not meet recommended dietary intake standards for fruits and vegetables.[21-23] Targeted patient and family education can help guide the patient in making healthier dietary choices. Structured lifestyle change programs have been shown to be beneficial in producing long-term weight loss of about 5–7% of baseline weight.[14,16] Thus, for an individual with a baseline weight of 165 lb (75 kg), a weight loss of 8–12 lb (3.5–5.5 kg) could prove beneficial.

Using a weight loss diet alone, however, is unlikely to produce long-term weight loss. Weight loss and its maintenance over time is enhanced by exercise and behavior modification. Thus, a planned exercise program tailored to the individual's physical capability, cognitive ability, and specific lifestyle circumstances is warranted. This is a primary focus of nutritional therapy for patients with DM and co-occurring psychiatric disorders. In a study of the dietary and exercise habits of patients with major affective disorders or schizophrenia, an average BMI of 29.6 (overweight) was observed. A large proportion of patients exhibited BMIs > 30 (obese). Exercise was reported to occur two or fewer times per week, indicating that these patients are less active than other persons of the same age. Among those who did report exercise activities, walking was the most popular activity noted.[5] The establishment of walking or exercise groups for individuals with serious mental illness can enhance physical activity levels, improve health self-perceptions, and facilitate social interactions that are part of a true psychosocial rehabilitation program.

Psychotropic medications, diabetes mellitus, and nutritional interventions

Many psychotropic medications increase weight and, for this reason alone, often lead to non-adherence. Mechanisms of weight gain are varied and may include decreased caloric utilization due to sedation, increased thirst and the subsequent intake of high-calorie beverages, increased appetite, and carbohydrate-craving associated with serotonin receptor blockade and histamine receptor antagonism.[24] Most of the weight gained while using various psychotropic medications has been observed to be fat weight and usually results not so much from an increase in overall quantity of intake but from a shift towards a greater proportion of high-calorie foods and beverages, particularly sugared carbonated beverages.[25]

Certain psychotropic medications, most notably the antipsychotic drugs, and especially the second-generation, or atypical, antipsychotics (SGAs) may place individuals at increased risk for obesity, insulin resistance, diabetes, high cholesterol, and, in certain cases, diabetic ketoacidosis.[4,26] For example, Allison et al assessed the likelihood of weight gain associated with the use of antipsychotic medications.[27] Controlling for gender and use of antipsychotics, the authors reported that weight gain was related to poor quality of life and reduced well-being and vitality. In a large VA study, the diabetes risk was highest for clozapine (hazard ratio [HR] = 1.57) and olanzapine (HR = 1.15); the diabetes risks for quetiapine (HR = 1.20) and risperidone (HR = 1.01) were not significantly different from that for conventional antipsychotics.[28]

Medications identified most likely to induce weight gain (Table 8.2) include the mood stabilizers, antipsychotics, especially clozapine, olanzapine, and phenothiazines, monoamine oxidase (MAO) inhibitors (isocarboxazid, phenelzine, and tranylcypromine), and among the newer antidepressants, mirtazapine and paroxetine.[29] For example, valproic acid, a mood stabilizer and anticonvulsant, has been associated with weight gain, insulin resistance, and elevated plasma insulin levels,[24] particularly in adult women. This significant weight gain is often associated with increased serum leptin levels. Increased serum leptin levels are associated with human obesity, and it has been suggested that obesity is a state of leptin resistance. Similarly, lithium

Table 8.2 Risk of weight gain associated with psychotropic medications

Drug category	Weight gain (kg)	Physical symptoms	Management
Antipsychotics	0.04–6.3	Constipation; dry mouth	Consider medication switch; encourage water as fluid of choice; high dietary fiber intake
Mood stabilizers	4–7	Increased fluid intake; preference for high-carbohydrate, high-fat foods	Avoid high calorie liquids (i.e. regular sodas, sugared drinks, alcohol); encourage water as fluid of choice
Anticonvulsants	4–7	Increased appetite and food intake	Reduce caloric intake
Antidepressants	2–4	Increased appetite and food intake; dry mouth	Monitor weight gain and dietary intake; adjust caloric intake; encourage water as fluid of choice
SSRIs	Minimal short-term; variable long-term	Increased appetite and food intake	Monitor weight gain and dietary intake; adjust caloric intake; consider medication switch
MAO inhibitors (phenelzine most common)	≥6.8	Enhances hypoglycemic effects of hypoglycemic drugs; increased thirst common	Avoid foods high in tyramine content; consume foods high in vitamin B_6; encourage water as fluid of choice

SSRIs, selective serotonin reuptake inhibitors; MAO, monoamine oxidase.

is associated with significant weight gain, insulin resistance, and hyperglycemia, and elevated serum leptin levels.

Coordinating medications for patients with co-occurring mental illness and diabetes creates a challenge and where possible the selection of psychotropic medications should avoid those that adversely affect weight gain or glycemic control. Usual strategies for the management of weight gain include consideration of change in medication to one that is more weight-neutral, increase inphysical activity, and review of dietary choices, as described above. Drug-holidays and dose tapering are strongly discouraged on the basis of concerns that patients' psychiatric illnesses may recur. For the treatment of depressive disorders, selective serotonin reuptake inhibitors (SSRIs) and atypical antidepressants (e.g. venlafaxine, duloxetine, and bupropion) show a relatively favorable short-term as well as long-term tolerability compared with older drugs (e.g. tricyclic antidepressants and MOA inhibitors). Therefore, clinicians are likely to prefer them in usual practice, especially among patients requiring maintenance treatment.

Factors that lead to enhanced adherence

For patients with mental illness, an intensification of treatment by the health care team when patients present for appointments is associated with improved diabetes outcomes. Diabetes knowledge scores of patients with mental illness are often lower than those reported among persons with type 2 DM from the general population. Dickerson et al recommend reducing these gaps in diabetes knowledge,[30] since the greater the level of diabetes-related knowledge the lower the level of perceived barriers to diabetes care. Specialized educational efforts should be appropriate to the cognitive level of the client. However, diabetes knowledge by itself does not significantly improve adherence to diet, glucose testing, or exercise programs.

Individuals who hold two important beliefs are more likely to engage in effective self-management behaviors than are those who do not hold these beliefs. The beliefs are:

- they consider their diabetes to be serious
- they believe that their actions make a difference.

An individual's self-confidence in making and maintaining a change is a significant predictor of later adherence. Balanced emotional support from family and friends is very helpful, as long as the patient does not perceive it to be intrusive or 'nagging', which can be counterproductive.

Comprehensive nutrition and exercise education programs have been shown to be effective weight management tools for patients with schizophrenia.[31] Education about nutrition and healthful food choices is necessary to assist patients with serious mental illness gain a sense of control over their diabetes with diet and exercise. Successful nutrition education and counseling efforts have included the use of simple 3-day dietary intake records to rapidly assess dietary adherence.[32] Consisting of two weekdays and one weekend day, the 3-day dietary record should include what foods were eaten when, as well as the approximate amounts. Encouraging patients to maintain records of physical activity can be combined with food records for simplicity (Figure 8.1). If the client is unable to maintain a record of foods eaten, a food 'recall' can be elicited at the time of visit.

Summary

The client with co-occurring DM and mental illness presents a unique set of challenges to health care providers. DM patients with mental illness have been noted to be more likely to have HbA_{1c} levels >8%, BMI >30 km/m^2, and serum triglyceride levels >400 mg/dl.[33] For MNT for DM to be effective, clients must be confident that they can make healthy lifestyle changes. A collaborative approach that includes the primary care physician, endocrinologist, psychiatrist, social worker, dietitian, and exercise physiologist,[15,34] with a structured program, has been found to be effective in helping this population of patients lose weight and improve glycemic control. Knowledge of the effects of psychotropic medications on body weight, lipid levels, and glucose tolerance are essential to appropriately address those factors that may adversely affect DM management, and to make reasonable choices regarding psychopharmacologic treatment. The contributions of a registered dietitian who regularly evaluates diet-related issues, provides ongoing counseling, and is an integral member of the health care team is invaluable in diabetes self-management in clients with mental illness.

Name:_____ Date:_____ Day of the week:_____

Food Diary

What did you eat and drink?	Amount?	What time of day?	How was it cooked?
Breakfast			
Snack			
Lunch			
Snack			
Dinner			
Snack			

Exercise Diary

☐   I walked _____ miles, _____ minutes, _____ steps _____

☐   I did other activities _____for _____minutes

Figure 8.1   Food and exercise diary.

References

1. National Institute of Diabetes and Digestive and Kidney Diseases. National Diabetes Statistics Fact Sheet: General information and national estimates on diabetes in the United States. Bethesda, MD: US Department of Health and Human Services, National Institute of Health, 2005.
2. Katon WJ, Von Korff M, Lin EHB et al. The pathways study: a randomized trial of collaborative care in patients with diabetes and depression. Arch Gen Psychiatry 2004; 61(10): 1042–9.

3. Lustman PJ, Gavard JA. Psychosocial aspects of diabetes in adult populations. National Diabetes Data Group National Institute of Health, National Institute of Diabetes and Digestive and Kidney Diseases. Diabetes in America, 2nd edn. NIH Publication No. 95-1468, 1995: 507–17.

4. Warren BH, Crews CK, Schulte MM. Managing patients with diabetes mellitus and mental health problems. Dis Manag Health Outcomes 2001; 9(3): 123–30.

5. Dixon LB, Wohlheiter K. Diabetes and mental illness: factors to keep in mind. Consultant 2003; 43(3): 337–40; 343–4.

6. Sernyak MJ, Leslie DL, Alarcon RD, Losonczy MF, Rosenheck R. Association of diabetes mellitus with use of atypical neuroleptics in the treatment of schizophrenia. Am J Psychiatry 2002; 159(4): 561–6.

7. Lin EHB, Katon W, Von Korff M et al. Relationship of depression and diabetes self-care, medication adherence, and preventive care. Diabetes Care 2004; 27(9): 2154–60.

8. Desai MM, Rosenheck RA, Druss BG, Perlin JB. Mental disorders and quality of diabetes care in the Veterans Health Administration. Am J Psychiatry 2002; 159(9): 1584–90.

9. Ciechanowski PS, Katon WJ, Russo JE, Hirsch IB. The relationship of depressive symptoms to symptom reporting, self-care, and glucose control in diabetes. Gen Hos Psychiatry 2003; 25: 246–52.

10. Musselman DL, Betan E, Larsen H, Phillips LS. Relationship of depression to diabetes types 1 and 2: epidemiology, biology, and treatment. Biol Psychiatry 2003; 54(3): 317–29.

11. Hwang SW, Bugeja AL. Barriers to appropriate diabetes management among homeless people in Toronto. CMAJ 2000; 163(2): 161–6.

12. Medicare Coverage Policy Decision: Duration and Frequency of the Medical Nutrition Therapy (MNT) Benefit (#CAG-00097N). http://frwebgate.access.gpo.gov

13. Franz MJ, Bantle JP, Beebe CA et al. American Diabetes Association position statement: evidence-based nutrition principles and recommendations for the treatment and prevention of diabetes and related complications. J Am Diet Assoc 2002; 102(1): 109–18.

14. Diabetes Prevention Program Research Group. Reduction in the incidence of type 2 diabetes with lifestyle intervention or metformin. N Engl J Med 2002; 346: 393–403.

15. Franz MJ, Monk A, Barry B et al. Effectiveness of medical nutrition therapy provided by dietitians in the management of non-insulin-dependent diabetes mellitus: a randomized, controlled clinical trial. J Am Diet Assoc 1995; 95(9): 1009–17.

16. Lemon CC, Lacey K, Lohse B et al. Outcomes monitoring of health, behavior and quality of life after nutrition intervention in adults with type 2 diabetes. J Am Diet Assoc 2004; 104(12): 1805–15.

17. Anderson JW, Randles KM, Kendall CWC, Jenkins DJA. Carbohydrate and fiber recommendations for individuals with diabetes: a quantitative assessment and meta-analysis of the evidence. J Am Coll Nutr 2004; 23(1): 5–17.

18. Institute of Medicine. Dietary Reference Intakes for Energy, Carbohydrate, Fiber, Fat, Fatty Acids, Cholesterol, Protein and Amino Acids. Washington, DC: The National Academies Press, 2002.

19. American Diabetes Association. Position Paper. Evidence-based nutrition principles and recommendations for the treatment and prevention of diabetes and related complications. Diabetes Care 2002; 25(Suppl 2).

20. Shogun NR, Pratt CA, Anderson A. Evaluation of nutrition education interventions for older adults: a proposed framework. J Am Diet Assoc 2004; 104: 58–69.
21. Brown S, Birtwistle J, Roe L, Thompson C. The unhealthy lifestyle of people with schizophrenia. Psychol Med 1999; 29(3): 697–701.
22. Wallace B, Tennant C. Nutrition and obesity in the chronic mentally ill. Aust N Z J Psychiatry 1998; 32(1): 82–5.
23. McCreadie RG, Scottish Schizophrenia Lifestyle Group. Diet, smoking and cardiovascular risk in people with schizophrenia: descriptive study. Br J Psychiatry 2003; 183: 534–9.
24. Haupt DW, Newcomer JW. Abnormalities in glucose regulation associated with mental illness and treatment. J Psychosom Res 2002; 53: 925–33.
25. Gothelf D, Falk B, Singer P et al. Weight gain associated with increased food intake and low habitual activity levels in male adolescent schizophrenic inpatients treated with olanzapine. Am J Psychiatry 2002; 159(6): 1055–7.
26. American Diabetes Association, American Psychiatric Association, American Association of Clinical Endocrinologists, North American Association for the Study of Obesity. Consensus Development Conference on Antipsychotic Drugs and Obesity and Diabetes. Diabetes Care 2004; 27(2): 596–601.
27. Allison DB, Mackell JA, McDonnell DD. The impact of weight gain on quality of life among persons with schizophrenia. Psychiatr Serv 2003; 54(4): 565–7.
28. Leslie DL, Rosenheck RA. Incidence of newly diagnosed diabetes attributable to atypical antipsychotic medications. Am J Psychiatry 2004; 161(9): 1709–11.
29. Ackerman S, Nolan LJ. Bodyweight gain induced by psychotropic drugs. Incidence, mechanisms and management. CNS Drugs 1998; 9(2): 135–51.
30. Dickerson FB, Goldberg RW, Brown CH et al. Diabetes knowledge among persons with serious mental illness and type 2 diabetes. Psychosomatics 2005; 46(5): 418–24.
31. Littrell KH. Obesity, diabetes, hyperlipidemia, and antipsychotic medications: breaking the link. Adv Stud Nurs 2004; 2(3): 101–9.
32. Leichter SB. Making outpatient care of diabetes more efficient: analyzing non-compliance. Clin Diabetes 2005; 23(4): 187–90.
33. Leichter SB, See Y. Problems that extend visit time and cost in diabetes care: 1. how depression may affect the efficacy and cost of care of diabetic patients. Clin Diabetes 2005; 23(2): 53–4.
34. Citrome L, Blonde L, Damatarca C. Metabolic issues in patients with severe mental illness. South Med J 2005; 98(7): 714–20.

Chapter 9

Impact of exercise on psychiatric disorders and diabetes mellitus

Neva J Kirk-Sanchez

Introduction

Lack of exercise and low levels of physical activity are risk factors for the development of many chronic diseases, including diabetes, depression, anxiety, and dementia. Conversely, increasing levels of physical activity and exercise can be an important intervention used to manage these diseases. Despite a wealth of evidence that most modes of exercise are effective in reducing symptoms and complications of diabetes and psychiatric disorders, exercise is infrequently used as a therapeutic modality. This chapter will review the evidence related to the benefits of exercise in reducing symptoms of diabetes mellitus (DM) and psychiatric disorders, including depression, anxiety, schizophrenia, and dementia. Information related to exercise prescription and improving adherence to exercise recommendations will also be discussed.

Physical activity and diabetes mellitus

Low levels of physical activity and a lifetime history of sedentary lifestyle are risk factors for the development of diabetes, pre-diabetes, and the metabolic syndrome.[1] Although exercise has been identified as a cornerstone for the prevention and management of DM, there is less attention paid to this mode of treatment than to pharmacological management or dietary modification.

Evidence identifying low levels of physical activity as a risk factor for DM has accumulated from multiple sources.[2] Studies of immigrant populations suggest that lifestyle changes related to movement to a new cultural and social environment may lead to an increasing prevalence of DM in these groups. In both of these cases, higher proportions of people with DM in these populations may be attributable to changes in the levels of habitual physical activity in groups immigrating from more rural, physically active societies to more urban, sedentary societies.[1] More direct evidence comes from longitudinal and retrospective epidemiologic studies showing that, in general, people with type 2 DM and impaired glucose tolerance are less physically active, and have been less active throughout their lifetimes, than people without type 2 DM.[1,2]

Clinical trials on groups of people both with and without risk factors for DM have indicated that physical activity can reduce the risk for developing DM and improve glucose tolerance and insulin sensitivity.[1–6] A meta-analysis of controlled clinical trials examining the impact of exercise on improving glycemic control in people with type 2 diabetes suggests that exercise training improves glycemic control to such an extent that it should decrease the risk of diabetic complications.[3] In the USA, the Diabetes Prevention Project demonstrated that a lifestyle intervention geared to decreasing body mass by 7% and performing 150 min/week of moderate physical activity decreased the incidence of diabetes by 58%.[4] The Finnish Diabetes Prevention Study also found a reduced risk of 58% compared with controls in the experimental group who received a lifestyle intervention with the goal of at least 5% reduction in body mass and 30 min/day of physical activity.[5] A 4-year follow-up of the Finnish Diabetes Prevention Study found a significant correlation between body mass and insulin sensitivity in participants.[6] These studies provide a wealth of evidence that exercise can be effective in improving glycemic control, thus reducing the risk for incidental DM and vascular complications in people who have DM.

Because DM is associated with dysfunction or failure of the cardiovascular system, the effect of DM on cardiovascular risk factors and symptoms should also be considered. DM is associated with hypertension, and it is well know that regular aerobic exercise can reduce blood pressure in people with hypertension. In addition, DM is associated with left ventricular diastolic dysfunction and impairment of endothelial vasodilator function, and both of these conditions may improve with moderate levels of aerobic exercise.[7] Finally, aerobic exercise is associated with reductions in body mass and intra-abdominal fat. Because higher body mass index (BMI) and abdominal adiposity are associated with both insulin resistance and coronary artery disease, weight loss accompanied by decreases in intra-abdominal fat may decrease the risk of micro- and macrovascular complications in people with DM.[7] Exercise may also lead to positive changes in lipid levels, but this may be related to reductions in body weight associated with exercise rather than the exercise itself.[8]

DM is a disease that is best controlled through self-management. Lifestyle behaviors, such as maintaining high levels of physical activity and appropriate diet and nutrition, are under the control of the patient with DM. However, people with DM must be educated about the benefits of exercise and diet in order to manage their disease appropriately. Most people with DM will benefit from loss of 5–10% of body weight. Too often, people with DM are given vague and generic instructions about the type, amount, and intensity of physical activity needed to manage their disease and reduce the risk of developing the vascular complications of DM. Unfortunately, people with DM are unable to adhere to recommendations and monitor progress if instructions are not clear and specific to their own needs and wishes. Health care practitioners who educate people with DM should be knowledgeable about specific recommendations, precautions, and contraindications of exercise and physical activity for the management of DM, and should be skilled in sharing this knowledge with the patients and clients with whom they interact.

Exercise therapy in diabetes mellitus management

Improvements in both glucose tolerance and glycemic control are positive outcomes of exercise for people with DM. Acute lowering of blood glucose levels is attributable to a decrease in hepatic glucose production accompanied by an increase in muscle glucose utilization and increased insulin sensitivity in peripheral muscles.[8] These favorable changes may be sustained for 12–24 hours after an exercise bout.[8] The acute effects of exercise training last for no more than 72 hours and are thought to reflect only the most recent exercise bout rather than exercise training.[8] Changes in glucose utilization, therefore, are transient and disappear a few days after an exercise bout. Therefore, long-term improvements seen with exercise training may reflect only the acute changes attributable to consecutive and continuing exercise bouts rather than a long-term improvement in glucose utilization or insulin resistance.

The magnitude of drop in blood glucose is related to the intensity and duration of exercise, pre-exercise levels, and the difficulty of the activity (Table 9.1). Most people with DM and obesity will show a decrease in blood glucose after moderate bouts of exercise; however, this effect is more variable in non-obese people with DM.[8] In people with hyperinsulinemia, high-intensity exercise may increase blood glucose, possibly due to a feedback mechanism that causes increased glucose production by the liver.[7,8] Thus, the evidence suggests that moderate exercise is the mode of choice in obese people with type II DM. There is less evidence supporting the benefit of moderate-intensity exercise for non-obese people with DM. Similarly, there is less evidence to support the benefits of high-intensity exercise, and high-intensity exercise may actually result in acute increases in blood glucose levels.[7,8]

Exercise for weight loss

Exercise results in mobilization in upper body and visceral fat, which are sources of free fatty acids leading to hyperglycemia in people with DM. In combination with adequate nutrition therapy, modest to moderate weight loss (10–15%) can improve glycemic control by multiple mechanisms. However, the American College of Sports Medicine (ACSM) recommendations point out that weight loss sufficient to cause positive effects in glycemic control would necessitate exercise at 50% of Vo_2 max, for 1 hour, 5 days/week, and sustained for years.[8] People with DM and obesity, especially in the presence of other chronic diseases, may be unable to attain and sustain this level of physical activity.[8,9]

Walking for diabetes mellitus management

Research studies investigating the impact of aerobic exercise on DM and glycemic control employ a number of modes of aerobic exercise, including walking or treadmill walking. As mentioned previously, some studies have found associations between habitual lifestyle physical activity

Table 9.1   Select examples of moderate and vigorous intensity physical activity

Moderate physical activity	Vigorous physical activity
Walking at a moderate to brisk pace – 3–4.5 mph on a level surface such as: • walking to class or work • walking for pleasure • walking the dog Walking downstairs or down a hill Racewalking less than 5 mph Using crutches Hiking	Racewalking or aerobic walking – 5 mph or faster Jogging or running Wheeling a wheelchair Walking/climbing briskly up a hill Backpacking
Bicycling 5–9 mph, level terrain Stationary using moderate effort	Bicycling more than 10 mph or bicycling on a steep uphill terrain Stationary bicycling – using vigorous effort
Low-impact aerobic dancing Water aerobics	High-impact aerobic dancing Step aerobics Water jogging
Light calisthenics Yoga Tai chi General home exercises, light or moderate effort, getting up and down from the floor Using a stair climbing machine at a light to moderate pace Using a rowing machine with moderate effort	Calisthenics – push-ups, pull-ups, vigorous effort Karate, judo, tae kwon do, jujitsu Jumping rope or jumping jacks Using a stair climbing machine at a fast pace Using a rowing machine – with vigorous effort Using an arm cycling machine – with vigorous effort
Weight training/bodybuilding using free weights or Nautilus/Universal type weights	Circuit weight training
Ballroom dancing, line dancing Folk or square dancing Modern dancing, disco Ballet	Any type of dancing – energetically Clogging
Recreational swimming Treading water with slow moderate effort	Swimming steady-paced laps Synchronized swimming Treading water with fast vigorous effort

US Department of Health and Human Services, Public Health Service, Centers for Disease Control and Prevention, National Center for Chronic Disease Prevention and Health Promotion, Division of Nutrition and Physical Activity. Reproduced with permission from *Promoting Physical Activity: A Guide for Community Action*. Champaign, IL: Human Kinetics, 1999.

such as walking and the risk for and management of type 2 DM.[2,10] An analysis of the National Health Interview Survey showed that walking more than 2 hours/week was associated with a 39% lower risk of death, and walking approximately 3–4 hours/week (30 min/day) was associated with a 50% lower risk of death in people with DM.[10] Furthermore, the protective benefit was greater for those walking at a moderate intensity rather than a higher intensity (see Table 9.1), and there was no more benefit provided by walking more than 3–4 hours/week.[10] It has been suggested that these protective benefits are greater than those achieved through other methods of diabetes management including pharmacologic strategies for blood pressure control, cholesterol-lowering, and strict glycemic control.[11] This is especially significant because moderate-intensity walking is an easily accessible activity, and may be more likely to be adhered to than prescribed exercise programs. The Health Professional's Follow-up Study also found a reduced risk of total mortality and cardiovascular disease in people with DM who were regular walkers, but in this case higher intensity activity (walking vs jogging vs running) was associated with even greater risk reductions.[12]

Resistance training

Resistance training is also beneficial in the management of DM and has been found to:

- enhance basal metabolism
- reduce visceral fat deposition
- improve insulin sensitivity and glycemic control
- increase muscle mass, strength, and endurance
- increase bone density
- decrease mobility impairment
- and decrease blood pressure.[9,13]

Additional psychological benefits include decreasing symptoms of anxiety and depression and improving self-efficacy.[13] Resistance training may be the mode of choice for very elderly, for morbidly obese adults with diabetes, or for those who have comorbid conditions which limit their ability to perform aerobic or weight-bearing exercises. For example, people with amputation, foot ulceration, or high fall risk may find strength training a safer and more feasible mode of exercise than aerobic exercise such as walking, cycling, or swimming.

Impact of exercise on psychiatric disorders

Results of cross-sectional and longitudinal studies indicate that exercise has a positive effect by reducing depression and anxiety and protecting against harmful consequences of stress.[14] This seems to be especially true in subclinical psychiatric disorders. In fact, evidence suggests that as little as one bout of exercise can result in significant changes in acute mood states.[15] Exercise may provide a valuable mode of non-pharmacologic intervention that also confers therapeutic social effects, and may be particularly useful for those patients for whom conventional psychotherapy or pharmacotherapy are less acceptable.[15–17]

People who are depressed tend to have lower levels of physical activity,[18,19] and evidence suggests that increasing activity levels and strength training seems to reduce symptoms of depression.[16,17] Physical activity also seems to reduce anxiety in people with high levels of anxiety and in people with more severe anxiety disorders such as panic disorder. Despite these facts, physical activity is underutilized in the treatment of psychological disorders such as depression and anxiety.[16,18]

Although few studies have examined the effect of exercise on people diagnosed with major depressive disorders, there is some evidence to support the benefit of both moderate- and vigorous-intensity physical activity[14,16] and of endurance training.[17–19] One study demonstrated that depression scores, as measured by the Beck Depression Inventory, were reduced after 9 weeks of vigorous activity,[18] and one meta-analysis has suggested that those patients with higher levels of depression had greater mental health improvements, with increased levels of physical activity.[19] In addition, some studies have found exercise to be as effective as psychotherapy in alleviating mild to moderate symptoms of depression.[18,20–22]

The mode of exercise that is most effective for alleviating depressive symptoms has also been studied, and it was found that aerobic exercise and strength and flexibility training had similar positive effects on symptoms of depression in both hospitalized[21] and non-hospitalized[22] patients. Additionally, it seems that a continuous (daily) moderate-intensity program has the same beneficial effect on symptoms of depression as intermittent, vigorous-intensity physical activity.[23]

Positive dose–response effects of leisure time and occupational physical activity have been illustrated by meta-analysis of both cross-sectional and prospective observational studies.[24] Evidence from this meta-analysis suggests that both moderate and vigorous exercise can reduce symptoms of depression. Finally, these positive effects were found with both aerobic and resistance training.[24] Dunn et al demonstrated in a randomized controlled trial comparing various exercise intensities that aerobic exercise at a dose of 17.5 kcal/kg/week is an effective treatment for major depressive disorder of mild to moderate severity,[25,26] and that exercise at lower intensities had effects similar to placebo. This translates to be approximately equivalent to the public health recommendations for exercise for all older adults of at least 30 min/day of moderate physical activity most days of the week. This study also found that energy expenditure was the important factor in reduction of symptoms, and that subjects who accumulated sufficient levels over 3 days and 5 days had similar positive effects.[26]

Impact of exercise on anxiety

Although few studies have examined the effect of exercise on anxiety disorders, one meta-analysis found that exercise is as efficacious as meditation or relaxation in reducing anxiety symptoms. In addition, findings suggest that aerobic exercise programs were more effective than weight-training or flexibility regimens. However, exercise needed to be 20–40 min/session for at least 10 weeks in order to be most effective, which suggests that moderate-duration exercise may be an important adjunct for the treatment of anxiety.[27]

For more severe anxiety disorders such as panic disorders, exercise was also found to be effective, although less effective than drug therapy, in alleviating symptoms.[28] This is significant, as many people with panic disorder falsely perceive exercise as detrimental, and thus abstain from physical activity due to fear.[16,17]

Exercise has also been shown to be an effective stand-alone treatment for panic disorder. One controlled trial compared a 10-week vigorous aerobic exercise program consisting of a progression from a 4-mile walk to a jog to pharmacologic management and placebo. This study demonstrated that exercise led to a significant decrease in symptoms, although pharmacologic management reduced symptoms more quickly and effectively.[28]

Impact of exercise on schizophrenia

People with schizophrenia are often taking medications associated with weight gain, poor glycemic control, and diabetes, and tend to have lower levels of fitness and physical activity.[29] In addition, people with schizophrenia also have symptoms of depression and anxiety. Therefore, exercise therapy and increasing physical activity may be a useful adjunct to traditional therapy, as it has the potential to reduce symptoms of depression and anxiety and may lower body mass and prevent excessive weight gain caused by the use of antipsychotic medications.

Although few studies have examined the effectiveness of exercise as an adjunct to the treatment of schizophrenia, those few have supported a positive association between physical activity and weight loss and increased fitness levels.[29] Benefits of exercise in this study also include decreased depression and anxiety and increased social interaction.[30] Exercise programs included treadmill walking and individually prescribed and supervised exercise programs.[30]

One small trial of exercise in patients with schizophrenia involved participation in individual exercise programs developed by exercise physiologists. A qualitative analysis of this program identified several themes. Involvement in the program improved the physical fitness of participants, and they felt positive about the social benefits of the group intervention while appreciating the individualized exercise prescription which allowed them to transition gradually to higher levels of physical activity. Additionally, the participants were eager to continue involvement in exercise and physical activity.[30]

Impact of exercise on dementia and cognitive impairment

Exercise in older adults with dementia has the potential to improve strength, movement, ability to perform activities of daily living, and cognitive status. Exercise programs have been found to be beneficial when used in the nursing home,[31,32] home,[33] or adult day-care environment.[34] Studies have demonstrated that a physical activity intervention, including a combination of aerobic activities, strength training, balance, and flexibility training, can reduce wandering, physical and verbal abusive behaviors, sleep disturbances, and the need for antipsychotic and hypnotic medications.[31] Physical activity can also have a positive effect on the functional mobility of people with moderate to severe dementia.[32-34] One study demonstrated that a walking program consisting of 30 minutes of assisted walking 3 days/week can have a positive effect on functional mobility, but must be combined with socialization in order to facilitate adherence and cooperation with the walking.[32] One study suggested that a strengthening program using elastic exercise bands may be an effective exercise modality for older adults with dementia in the day-care setting.[34] Elastic exercise bands may be the modality of choice for people with dementia, as there is less risk for injury than there might be when using free weights or exercise machines.

A meta-analysis of 30 selected trials of exercise in older adults with dementia provides evidence to support the effectiveness of exercise programs for improving strength, cardiovascular fitness, behavior, and cognition.[35] The average duration of training regimens was 23 weeks, and regimens were usually based on walking or combined walking with isotonic exercises.[35]

Facilitating physical activity in older adults with dementia can be a challenge, and impairments in reasoning and judgment often lead to poor adherence. Structured exercise training in the home or nursing home environment should include strength, endurance, flexibility, and balance training in conjunction with caregiver training, as this combination has been shown to be effective in increasing physical activity levels.[33]

Exercise training recommendations for people with diabetes mellitus and psychiatric disorders

People with psychiatric disorders have no specific contraindications for aerobic exercise, and exercise guidelines for the general population should be used to prescribe exercise programs. The ACSM[8] and the American Diabetes Association (ADA)[36] recommend that people with type 2 DM without significant complications or comorbidity accumulate at least 1000 kcal/week of physical activity.[8] This is similar to the recommendations derived from a technical review of 150 min/week of moderate-intensity aerobic activity.[37] This should include 3 non-consecutive days of physical activity, up to 5 days/week. Because the duration of insulin sensitivity after a single bout of exercise is not greater than 72 hours, time between successive sessions of physical activity should be less than 72 hours, or no more than 2 days between successive exercise bouts.[8,36,37] Because of the difficulties in balancing insulin levels in those with DM, it may be more helpful for people to engage in aerobic activity every day. In addition, patients with obesity may need to perform aerobic activity daily in order to balance nutrient intake and uptake for effective weight management.[8]

Just as for any person completing an exercise session, sessions should begin with a 10–15 minute period of warm-up and end with a 5–10 minute period of cool-down that includes lower-intensity aerobic exercises and flexibility exercises.[8] People who have not been exercising should start with 10–15 minutes of aerobic exercise daily and advance to at least 30 minutes of activity.[36] Because people with type 2 DM and those with psychiatric disorders generally have a low level of cardiovascular fitness, they should start exercise at a relatively low intensity (rating of perceived exertion of 10–12 or 40–60% Vo_2 max) and progress slowly. In addition, exercising at a lower level may improve adherence, as exertion levels are more comfortable than at higher levels. Finally, lower-intensity exercise will decrease the risk for musculoskeletal injury and foot problems in people with DM.[38] People with DM have a significant increase in the risk of cardiovascular disease, and in order to reduce the risk larger volumes of exercise may be necessary. The ADA recommends at least 4 hours/week of moderate to vigorous activity in order to reduce cardiovascular risk.[36,37]

Weight loss is an important strategy in DM management and for people taking some drugs to manage psychiatric disorders. Weight loss generally requires combinations of diet and exercise. However, the volume of exercise needed to sustain weight loss is higher than that needed to sustain glycemic control. ADA recommendations emphasize that a much longer duration of moderate-intensity exercise, approximately 1 hour of exercise 7 days/week, is necessary to lose weight.[37,39]

Thus, the frequency, intensity, and sequencing of exercise should be modified according to the desired outcomes. The minimum effective dose of aerobic exercise appears to be moderate-intensity exercise for 30 consecutive minutes, at least three times a week, with no more than 2 days between exercise bouts. More frequent, longer-duration, or higher-intensity exercise is necessary if weight loss or reduction of cardiovascular risk are the desired outcomes.

Whether or not the desired outcome includes significant weight loss, adherence to an aerobic activity program is challenging for many people. People with DM and/or psychiatric disorders should perform aerobic activities which are low to moderate intensity, are easily gauged in their intensity, are generally approved by the person, are familiar, and require little skill.[36–38] Exercise should use large muscle groups such as the trunk, hips, and shoulders and be rhythmic and sustainable in nature to be the most effective. For this reason, walking is often the aerobic activity of choice. Weight-bearing activities such as walking or jogging, however, may lead to problems in the foot and lower extremity for some people with DM.[38] For people with diabetic peripheral neuropathy, swimming or stationary biking may be a better choice, as these are not weight-bearing activities.[37] The health care practitioner should use knowledge of contraindications, a patient's medical condition including existing and potential complications of diabetes, and a knowledge about risks and benefits of exercise to assist the patients in developing an exercise program that is safe, feasible, and likely to be adhered to. Guidelines for prescription of aerobic exercise in patients with diabetes and psychiatric disorders are found in Table 9.2. Absolute and relative contraindications to exercise participation are found in Table 9.3. Examples of both moderate and vigorous intensity exercise are found in Table 9.1.

Resistance training has also been found to be an effective means of lowering blood glucose and improving glycemic control.[2,9,10] Resistance training also has positive effects for lowering symptoms of depression and anxiety, reducing symptoms of schizophrenia, and improving cognitive and physical status in people with dementia. The ACSM recommends that resistance training should be performed at least 2 days/week, when feasible.[8] The ACSM recommends that resistance training consists of 8–10 exercises using large muscle groups with a minimum of 10–15 repetitions to near fatigue.[8] The ADA further recommends that weight-training programs are performed with low weights and high repetitions, for all major muscle groups at least three times per week at a weight than cannot be lifted more than 8–10 times.[36,37] The ADA[36] and the ACSM[8] further emphasize that, in order to maximize health benefit and minimize risk for injury, resistance training should initially be supervised by an exercise specialist.

Although exercise guidelines are available, more research is needed to determine the effects of specific resistance training regimens on glycemic control in people with DM. One study combined aerobic and resistance training in a circuit training format, and found that participants improved functional capacity, lean body mass, strength, and most importantly glycemic control in people with type 2 DM.[40] Existing evidence therefore suggests that circuit training, using a combination of

Table 9.2   Exercise guidelines/recommendations for people with diabetes and psychiatric disorders

Training	Exercise parameters
Aerobic training	
Mode	Walking, swimming, or biking at moderate intensity
Duration	150 min/week
Intensity	40–60% of Vo_2 max
Frequency	5–6 times weekly, no more than 2 days between exercise sessions
Resistance training	
Mode	Large muscle groups
	Using free weights, Nautilus or Universal equipment, or elastic exercise bands
	Dynamic lifting or pulling tasks
	Slow velocity during eccentric phase
Intensity	1–2 sets of 8–15 repetitions
	6–8 exercise groups
	40–60% of 1 rep-max
Frequency	1–2 times weekly

moderate-intensity aerobic activity such as walking or cycling, and a resistance training regimen, using large muscle groups, relatively high repetitions, and relatively low resistance, may be the most beneficial and feasible regimen to manage DM and may have positive effects for people with psychiatric disorders. Guidelines for prescription of resistance training for people with DM and resistance training are found in Table 9.3.[38]

The Surgeon's Report on Physical Activity recommendations for physical activity[41] also include both flexibility exercises and balance exercises as important components of physical activity programs in all groups of people, including those with diabetes. Therefore, flexibility exercises and balance exercises should be incorporated into a well-rounded exercise program 2–3 days/week.

Precautions and contraindications

Both the ACSM[8] and the ADA[42] have recommended that individuals with type 2 DM should undergo an exercise stress test prior to initiating a moderate-intensity exercise program. This allows an individualized

Table 9.3 Precautions and contraindications for exercise training (ACSM guidelines for exercise testing and prescription)

Absolute contraindications for exercise training:
- Recent change in resting ECG that has not been evaluated or managed
- Unstable angina, left CAD, or cardiac symptoms provoked by exercise training
- Uncontrolled congestive heart failure
- Uncontrolled arrhythmias causing symptoms or hemodynamic insufficiency
- Severe symptomatic aortic stenosis
- Large or expanding aortic aneurysm
- Acute myocarditis or pericarditis
- Acute DVT or PE or infarction
- Acute retinal disorder or recent ophthalmic surgery
- Acute or inadequately controlled renal failure
- Acute infections

Relative contraindications for exercise training:
- Fasting blood glucose > 300 mg/dl or > 250 mg/dl with ketone bodies
- Uncontrolled hypertension, systolic > 200 mmHg and/or diastolic > 110 mmHg
- Autonomic neuropathy with exertional hypotension
- Severe stenotic valve disease
- Unstable arrhythmias
- Ventricular aneurysm
- Electrolyte abnormalities
- Uncontrolled COPD or RLD
- Recent cerebral or subdural hemorrhage or cerebral aneurysm
- Unstable or progressive neurologic disease
- Uncontrolled systemic disease (metabolic or infectious diseases)
- Neuromuscular, musculoskeletal, or rheumatoid disorders that are exacerbated by exercise
- Complicated pregnancy
- Unstable, injured, or acutely inflamed joints, tendons, or ligaments
- Fractures within last 6 weeks to 6 months
- Large abdominal or inguinal hernias or hemorrhoids

ACSM, American College of Sports Medicine; ECG, electrocardiogram; CAD, coronary artery disease; DVT, deep vein thrombosis; PE, pulmonary embolism; COPD, chronic obstructive pulmonary disease; RLD, restrictive lung disease.

exercise prescription based on blood pressure response, and maximal heart rate. The prevalence of cardiac ischemia and silent ischemia, as well as abnormal blood pressure responses, is higher in people with diabetes.[7,8] In addition, problems associated with retinal neuropathy, peripheral neuropathy, and autonomic neuropathy should be identified through a thorough physical examination and cardiac stress test.[8,42] The ADA recommendation asserts that maximal exercise testing could be 'considered' in all diabetic individuals, but highlights the fact that this testing might be cost prohibitive.[37] The most recent recommendation

Table 9.4   Indications for exercise ECG testing prior to initiation of vigorous exercise program[a]

Presence of any of the factors below indicates a need for pre-exercise testing:
- Known or suspected CAD
- Type 2 DM of more than 10 years' duration
- Age over 35 years
- Any additional risk factors for CAD
- Microvascular disease
- Peripheral vascular disease
- Autonomic neuropathy

ECG, electrocardiogram; CAD, coronary artery disease; DM, diabetes mellitus.

[a]Patients who do not undergo exercise ECG testing should perform only light to moderate exercise programs.

Adapted from Schneider and Shindler.[42]

suggests that maximal exercise testing should be strongly considered in those who are beginning a program of physical activity more intense than brisk walking.[37,42] This modification limits the need for an exercise stress test in those who are undergoing lifestyle intervention programs that do not include strenuous physical activity. Criteria for exercise testing can be found in Table 9.4.

Individuals with DM may develop autonomic neuropathy and have an abnormal heart rate response to exercise. It is imperative that individuals with autonomic neuropathy undergo an exercise stress test before engaging in exercise more intense than that to which they are accustomed.[37,41] In addition, the Borg Rating of Perceived Exertion (RPE) scale should be used to gauge exercise intensity.[8,37,41] Individuals with DM and autonomic neuropathy should be trained in the appropriate use of the RPE scale to monitor and progress the intensity of the exercise program.

Other vascular complications associated with DM should be considered when prescribing an exercise program. For example, vigorous aerobic or resistance exercise may be contraindicated for those with retinopathy, and patients should abstain from exercise for 3–6 months after laser photocoagulation.[37] Weight-bearing exercise may be contraindicated in those with peripheral neuropathy, due to the risk of injury to the foot or skin breakdown. Instead, individuals with severe peripheral neuropathy should engage in swimming, bicycling, or arm exercises.[37,41]

Regardless of the mode of exercise performed, people with DM should take care to reduce the risk for hypoglycemia associated with exercise. Blood glucose monitoring should occur prior to exercising, and exercise should not be initiated if blood glucose levels are < 100 mg/dl. This is especially important in those who are taking insulin, and in fact, most recent recommendations state that carbohydrate supplementation is generally unnecessary in those treated only with diet, metformin, glucosidase inhibitors, or thiazolidinediones, but may be necessary in those using insulin for DM management.[8,37] In addition, insulin or glucose-reducing oral medications should be ingested not less than 1 hour prior to exercise. Insulin should not be injected into muscles that are being heavily utilized in the exercise regimen. For those initiating an exercise regimen, insulin or oral hypoglycemic agent doses may need to be adjusted.[8,37] Additionally, monitoring of blood glucose levels may be necessary before, after, and several hours after an exercise session, especially for people who take insulin or insulin secretagogues.[8,36,37] Ingestion of additional carbohydrate and fluids is only necessary if exercise is of high intensity or long duration (60–90 minutes).[8,37]

Adherence to exercise by people with diabetes mellitus and psychiatric disorders

In studies examining the role of exercise training in reducing symptoms of depression, only 50% of individuals, both with and without major depression, who initiated exercise programs completed the programs.[15] Similar trends of poor adherence are seen in people with diabetes.[36] Factors related to exercise adherence have been identified as attitudes towards the benefits of exercise, self-efficacy and behavioral control, exercise intention, past and recent involvement in physical activity, physical condition, knowledge about exercise, and perceived social support.[36,37] It is important for people with depression or DM to complete an adequate trial of exercise in order to assess the effectiveness in alleviating symptoms. Therefore, it is imperative that clinicians understand and utilize methods to encourage and facilitate adherence to prescribed exercise regimens.

Two models commonly used to help health educators provide information about physical activity and exercise programs are the self-efficacy or social learning model[43] and the transtheoretical model of behavioral change.[44]

The transtheoretical model of behavioral change suggests that persons are at different levels of cognitive readiness to adopt or maintain a particular health behavior, such as exercise.[44] This model suggests that there are five stages of readiness: precontemplation, contemplation, preparation, action, and maintenance. These stages can be assessed by the responses to questions related to whether or not patients are thinking about initiating an exercise program in the next 6 months (contemplation and preparation), whether they are actually participating in an exercise program (action) and, if so, whether they have been exercising for more than 6 months (maintenance).[44] Intervention and education related to exercise should take into account the current stage of readiness and be modified to assist the patient in moving through these stages.

Self-efficacy is the belief in one's capabilities to execute a specific behavior or action to satisfy the demands of the situation. Self-efficacy is theorized to influence the behavior or tasks that individuals choose to perform, the effort exerted in completing the tasks, and the degree of persistence in the face of aversive stimuli such as failure to adequately complete the task or perform the behavior.[43] Perception of personal self-efficacy related to exercise is an important predictor of adherence to prescribed exercise behaviors. In fact, the best predictor of adherence to exercise programs is past success in performing exercises. Health care practitioners can influence an individual's exercise self-efficacy in several ways, including emphasizing performance attainments, providing opportunities for vicarious experience, using verbal persuasion to encourage and coach patients and clients, and being alert to states of anxiety that may occur during exercise sessions.

Practitioners can emphasize performance attainment by questioning individuals explicitly about past successes, and discussing the factors that may have led to successful exercise experiences in the past. Using support groups to encourage others to share their positive experiences with exercise can also improve self-efficacy. Practitioners should be able to offer positive feedback in the form of verbal praise for small successes in adherence to exercise and should be able to help individuals problem-solve about factors related to less successful exercise experiences. Finally, states of anxiety experienced during an exercise session can lead to poorer perceptions of self-efficacy. Practitioners can promote calm and reduce anxiety by modifying the exercise environment and specifically addressing stressors related to exercise.

Table 9.5 Strategies to improve adherence for individuals at different stages of readiness for adoption of exercise behaviors

Exercise stage of readiness
- Precontemplation stage – individual is not thinking about exercise
- Contemplation stage – individual is thinking about exercise, but is not planning on initiating an exercise program in the next 6 months
- Preparation stage – individual is thinking about initiating an exercise program in the next 6 months
- Action stage – individual has initiated an exercise program, but has not been sustaining exercise for 6 months
- Maintenance stage – individual has been regularly exercising for ≥6 months

Precontemplation stage	Goal:	inform individual about benefits of exercise in disease management and prevention
	•	Describe the benefits of exercise using positive wording,emphasizing the potential long-term benefits rather than the negative consequences of not exercising
	•	Emphasize the social and psychological benefits as well as the health benefits of exercise programs
Contemplation and preparation stages	Goal:	increase self-efficacy related to exercise
	•	Describe the benefits of exercise using positive wording, emphasizing the potential long-term benefits rather than the negative consequences of not exercising
	•	Emphasize the social and psychological benefits as well as the health benefits of exercise programs
	•	Assure the patient that exercise does not need to be strenuous or painful to have a benefit; emphasize lifestyle interventions
	•	Explain to individuals that they will have the assistance of a health care practitioner to set up an exercise program that meets their needs and wishes
Action stage	Goal:	specific exercise prescription
	•	Provide specific information regarding mode, duration, intensity, and frequency of exercise
	•	Provide specific information about progression of exercises
	•	Explain to the individual precautions, specifically those related to diabetes such as foot care and glycemic control
	•	Assist the individual in goal setting and monitoring of progress
Maintenance stage	Goal:	injury prevention and progression of intensity of exercise
	•	Check to make sure the individual is using exercise equipment, including footwear, appropriately
	•	Assist the individual in setting attainable, measurable goals, and monitor progress

Table 9.5   Continued

- Encourage adherence strategies such as using an exercise schedule or an exercise partner
- Encourage self-rewards and incentives
- Identify different exercise activities to prevent boredom and burnout
- Assure the individual that backsliding is not failure, and encourage those who experience temporary lapses in exercise behaviors to continue working toward success

Adapterd from Marrero.[36]

Studies of adherence to exercise programs often use a social learning model that identifies barriers to exercise such as lack of skill, lack of support, and lack of access. Another key point in the social learning model is the benefit of environmental cues to action that facilitate adherence to health-related behaviors. In the context of the social learning model, prescribing an exercise program that is individualized to match the physical ability, attitude, belief, and lifestyle of a diabetic patient may improve adherence by increasing the expectations of success. Table 9.5 summarizes strategies to encourage adherence to exercise programs by promoting self-efficacy at differing stages of exercise readiness according to the transtheoretical model.[36,37]

Summary

This chapter has reviewed the benefits of lifestyle physical activity, aerobic exercise, and resistance training for people with DM and psychiatric disorders. The benefits of exercise and physical activity for this population are clear. Assisting people to develop and implement an exercise and physical activity regimen that is safe, feasible, and likely to be adhered to is a difficult task for the health care practitioner. However, a specific exercise prescription based on established guidelines, and support for good adherence to the program can assist people with DM and psychiatric disorders to be successful in improving health behaviors related to exercise and physical activity. These habits and behaviors can provide important therapeutic benefits in the management of DM and psychiatric disorders.

References

1. Ivy JL. Exercise physiology and adaptations to training. In: Ruderman N, Devlin JT, Schneider SH, Kriska A, eds. Handbook of Exercise in Diabetes, 2nd edn. Alexandria, VA: American Diabetes Association, 2002: 23–63.

2. Hawley JA. Exercise as a therapeutic intervention for the prevention and treatment of insulin resistance. Diabetes Metab Res Rev 2004; 20: 383–93.

3. Boule NG, Haddad E, Kenny GP, Wells GA, Sigal RJ. Effects of exercise on glycemic control and body mass in type 2 diabetes mellitus: a meta-analysis of controlled clinical trials. JAMA 2001; 286: 1218–27.

4. Diabetes Prevention Program Research Group. Reduction in the incidence of type 2 diabetes with lifestyle intervention or metformin. N Engl J Med 2002; 46(6): 393–403.

5. Tuomilehto J, Lindstrom J, Ericsson JG et al. Prevention of type 2 diabetes mellitus by changes in lifestyle among subjects with impaired glucose tolerance. N Engl J Med 2001; 344(18): 1343–50.

6. Uusitupa M, Lindi V, Louheranta A et al. Long-term improvement in insulin sensitivity by changing lifestyles of people with impaired glucose tolerance: 4-year results from the Finnish Diabetes Prevention Study. Diabetes 2003; 52: 2532–8.

7. Stewart KJ. Exercise training and the cardiovascular consequences of type 2 diabetes and hypertension: plausible mechanisms for improving cardiovascular health. JAMA 2002; 299(13): 1622–31.

8. American College of Sports Medicine Position Stand. Exercise and type II diabetes. Med Sci Sports Exer 2000; 32: 1345–60.

9. Willey KA, Fiatarone-Singh MA. Battling insulin resistance in elderly obese people with type 2 diabetes: bring on the heavy weights. Diabetes Care 2000; 26(5): 1580–8.

10. Gregg EW, Gerzoff RB, Caspersin EJ et al. Relationship of walking to mortality among US adults with diabetes. Arch Intern Med 2003; 164: 1440–7.

11. Hu FB. Walking. The best medicine for diabetes? Arch Intern Med 2003; 163: 1397–8.

12. Tanasescu M, Leitzmann MF, Rimm EB, Hu FB. Physical activity in relation to cardiovascular disease and total mortality among men with type 2 diabetes. Circulation 2003; 107: 2435–9.

13. Pollock ML, Franklin BA, Balady GJ et al. Resistance exercise in individuals with and without cardiovascular disease: benefits, rationale, safety, and prescription. Circulation 2000; 101: 828–33.

14. Salmon P. Effects of physical exercise on anxiety, depression, and sensitivity to stress: a unifying theory. Clin Psychol Rev 2001; 20(1): 33–61.

15. Yeung RR. The acute effects of exercise on mood state. J Psychosom Res 1996; 40(2): 123–41.

16. Paluska SA, Schwenk TL. Physical activity and mental health: current concepts. Sports Med 2000; 29(3): 167–80.

17. Meyer T, Broocks A. Therapeutic impact of exercise on psychiatric diseases: Guidelines for exercise testing and prescription. Sports Med 2000; 30(4): 269–79.

18. Martinsen EW, Medhaus A, Sandvik L. Effects of exercise on depression: a controlled study. Br Med J (Clin Res Ed) 1985; 291: 109.

19. North TC, McCullagh P, Tran AV. Effect of exercise on depression. Exerc Sport Sci Rev 1990; 18: 379–415.

20. Martinsen EW. Benefits of exercise for the treatment of depression. Sports Med 1990; 9(6): 380–9.

21. Martinsen EW, Hoffart A, Solberg O. Comparing aerobic with nonaerobic forms of exercise in the treatment of clinical depression: a randomized trial. Compr Psychiatry 1989; 30(4): 324–31.

22. Doyne EJ, Ossip-Klein DJ, Bowman ED et al. Running versus weightlifting in the treatment of depression. J Consult Clin Psychol 1987; 55(5): 748–54.

23. Dunn AL, Marcus BH, Kambert JB et al. Comparison of lifestyle and structured interventions to increase physical activity and cardiorespiratory fitness: a randomized trial. JAMA 1999; 281(4): 327–34.

24. Dunn AL, Trivedi MH, O'Neal HA. Physical activity dose–response effects on outcomes of depression and anxiety. Med Sci Sports Exerc 2001; 33(6 Suppl): S587–97.

25. Dunn AL, Trivedi MH, Kampert JB, Clark CG, Chambliss HO. The DOSE study: A clinical trial to examine efficacy and dose reponse of exercise as treatment for depression. Control Clin Trials 2002; 23(5): 584–603.

26. Dunn AL, Trivedi MH, Kampert JB, Clark CG, Chambliss HO. Exercise treatment for depression: efficacy and dose response. Am J Prev Med 2005; 28(1): 1–8.

27. Petruzzello SJ, Landers DM, Hatfield BD et al. A meta-analysis of the anxiety reducing effects of acute and chronic exercise. Sports Med 1991; 11(3): 143–82.

28. Broocks A, Bandelow B, Pekrun G et al. Comparison of aerobic exercise, clomipramine, and placebo in the treatment of panic disorder. Am J Psychiatry 1998; 155(5): 603–9.

29. Beebe LH, Tian L, Morris N et al. Effects of exercise on mental and physical health parameters of persons with schizophrenia. Issues Mental Health Nurs 2005; 26: 661–76.

30. Fogarty M, Happell B. Exploring the benefits of an exercise program for people with schizophrenia: a qualitative study. Issues Ment Health Nurs 2005; 26: 341–51.

31. Landi F, Russo A, Bernabie R. Physical activity and behavior in the elderly: a pilot study. Arch Gerontol Geriatr Suppl 2004; 9: 235–41.

32. Tappen RM, Roach KE, Applegate EB, Stowell P. Effect of a combined walking and conversation intervention on functional mobility of nursing home residents with Alzheimer disease. Alzheimer Dis Assoc Disord 2000; 14(4): 196–201.

33. Teri L, McCurry SM, Buchner DM et al. Exercise and activity level in Alzheimer's disease: a potential treatment focus. J Rehab Res Develop 1998; 35(4): 411–19.

34. Thomas VS, Hageman PA. Can neuromuscular strength and function in people with dementia be rehabilitated using resistance-exercise training? Results from a preliminary intervention study. J Gerontol A Biol Sci Med Sci 2003; 58(8): 746–51.

35. Heyn P, Abreu BC, Ottenbacher KJ. The effects of exercise training on elderly persons with cognitive impairment and dementia: a meta-analysis. Arch Phys Med Rehabil 2005; 85: 1694–704.

36. Marrero DG. Initiation and maintenance of exercise in patients with diabetes. In: Ruderman N, Devlin JT, Schneider SH, Kriska A, eds. Handbook of Exercise in Diabetes, 2nd edn. Alexandria, VA: American Diabetes Association, 2002: 289–310.

37. Sigal RJ, Kenny GP, Wasserman DH, Castaneda-Sceppa C. Physical activity/exercise and type 2 diabetes. Diabetes Care 2004; 27(10): 2518–39.

38. Gordon NF. The exercise prescription. In: Ruderman N, Devlin JT, Schneider SH, Kriska A, eds. Handbook of Exercise in Diabetes, 2nd edn. Alexandria, VA: American Diabetes Association, 2002: 269–88.

39. Wing RR. Exercise and weight control. In: Ruderman N, Devlin JT, Schneider SH, Kriska A, eds. Handbook of Exercise in Diabetes, 2nd edn. Alexandria, VA: American Diabetes Association, 2002: 355–76.

40. Maiorana A, O'Driscoll G, Goodman C, Taylor R, Green D. Combined aerobic and resistance exercise improves glycemic control and fitness in type 2 diabetes. Diabetes Res Clin Pract 2002; 56: 115–23.

41. US Department of Health and Human Services. Physical Activity and Health: A Report of the Surgeon General. Atlanta, GA: US Department of Health and Human Services, Centers for Disease Control and Prevention, National Center for Chronic Disease Prevention and Health Promotion, 1996.

42. Schneider SH, Shindler D. Application of the American Diabetes Associations's Guidelines for the evaluation of the diabetic patient before recommending an exercise program. In: Ruderman N, Devlin JT, Schneider SH, Kriska A, eds. Handbook of Exercise in Diabetes, 2nd edn. Alexandria, VA: American Diabetes Association, 2002: 253–68.

43. Bandura A. Social Foundations of Thought and Action. Englewood Cliffs, NJ: Prentice Hall, 1986.

44. Prochaska JO, Velicer WF. The transtheoretical model of health behavior change. Am J Health Promot 1997; 12: 38–48.

Chapter 10

Psychopharmacologic treatment of psychiatric disorders in patients with diabetes mellitus: clinical considerations and options

Jose A Rey

Introduction

The purpose of this chapter is to provide the practitioner with a selection of potential treatment options for the care of depression, bipolar disorder, the anxiety disorders, insomnia, and schizophrenia in patients who also have comorbid diabetes mellitus (DM) or where DM risk is a factor in medication selection. A greater detailed discussion regarding the diagnostics, risk factors, and specific metabolic relationships of the various psychiatric illnesses as well as the metabolic effects of the antipsychotics is provided elsewhere in this book and therefore only briefly addressed in this chapter. Although no particular psychotropic medication is specifically contraindicated in persons with DM, certain agents probably carry a higher risk for exacerbating this chronic endocrinologic and metabolic disorder. Some psychotropics may increase plasma glucose levels, increase glycosylated hemoglobin A_{1c} (HbA_{1c}), or cause insulin resistance vs other psychotropics that may cause hypoglycemia or increase insulin sensitivity. The negative effects of some psychotropics on diabetic control may have more to do with appetite stimulation or weight gain than a direct effect on glucose and insulin physiology. These changes in glucose response may be short-term reactions to the psychotropic drug. At other times, effects may only occur after long-term exposure to the agent, making it difficult to discern the influence of the medication from the possible progression of the underlying diabetes pathology. Either way, the person with DM and a comorbid psychiatric illness must receive a higher level of monitoring for both the clinical and laboratory outcomes of their DM and glycemic control and for the psychiatric management of the targeted mental illness which may be secondary to, or exacerbated by, the person's DM.

Depressive disorders

Previous chapters have described the frequent co-occurrence of DM and depressive disorders. Unfortunately, there is a paucity of literature evaluating the efficacy of antidepressants in the treatment of the depressed patient with DM. In discussing the impact of the antidepressants on DM and glycemic control, the practitioner must bear in mind that the desired goal of improvement in the patient's mood state may also directly, or indirectly, lead to improvement in diabetic control through increased insulin sensitivity, change in appetite and reduction in weight, decreased stress and cortisol-related hyperglycemia, improvement in adherence to medication regimens, and overall improvement in quality of life. Therefore it is difficult to fully assess the impact of an antidepressant, or any psychotropic, on the depressed patient's diabetic control due to the possible non-pharmacologic influences. Laboratory studies have provided some evidence of the ability of certain antidepressants to increase or decrease certain diabetic parameters, but this chapter will be largely referring to clinical studies that assessed these parameters in depressed patients or to studies that reported changes in glycemic parameters and weight in non-diabetic patients and use these reports, or animal study data when necessary, as supplemental support of recommendations.

Antidepressants

No particular antidepressant is contraindicated in the treatment of depression in persons with DM, and data regarding the class' impact on diabetic management is mixed. This may be due to subclass differences in pharmacologic characteristics such as targeted neurotransmitter or receptor effects. The efficacy of some antidepressants in treating symptoms of depression in persons with DM has been proven.[1-3] The practitioner should note that other antidepressants are also well established as having the added benefit of improving the symptoms of diabetic neuropathy, even in non-depressed patients with this painful syndrome.[4,5] This may prompt the practitioner to consider an antidepressant that could address this painful syndrome for a patient with coexisting depression and thus minimize the need for multiple drug treatment regimens.

Tricyclic antidepressants

The tricyclic antidepressants (TCAs) have been available since the 1950s with the introduction of imipramine. It should be noted that we often named our older psychotropics based on their molecular structure: i.e. the three-ring structure of a TCA gives it the name. Today, if imipramine was discovered and developed as an antidepressant, it would be called, or labeled, a serotonin–norepinephrine reuptake inhibitor (SNRI), just as we label venlafaxine or duloxetine. Some TCAs are more potent at the inhibition of serotonin (5-hydroxytryptamine or 5-HT) reuptake (e.g. clomipramine, imipramine), some are relatively balanced in their reuptake inhibition of these two neurotransmitters (e.g. doxepin, trimipramine), and others are more potent at inhibiting the reuptake of norepinephrine (NE), such as desipramine or nortriptyline.[6] These neurotransmitter profiles and the varied other receptor antagonism that the TCAs possess may influence, in both positive and negative ways, the management of the person with diabetes and depression. For example, a clinical study by Lustman et al reported the efficacy of nortriptyline in treating depression in a diabetic population; however, this study also revealed that this agent may worsen diabetic laboratory parameters and cause weight gain.[1]

Because of the significant adverse-effect profile of the TCAs, even in a non-diabetic and otherwise healthy population, the practice of prescribing TCAs has diminished. This subclass of antidepressants is commonly considered to be second- or third-line agents for the treatment of depression, not for lack of efficacy, but due to potential risks for cardiac toxicities and other problematic adverse effects such as anticholinergic effects, orthostasis, and sedation.[7] These adverse effects may be even more problematic in diabetic patients, who may also have other comorbid disorders such as cardiovascular disease. The weight gain associated with TCAs has been established for many years through clinical experience and research.[7,8] Glycemic control may actually fluctuate between hypoglycemia and hyperglycemia, and these outcomes may be related to the length of exposure to these antidepressants along with the neurotransmitter profile of the TCA being either more serotonergic or more noradrenergic in nature and the level of antihistamine effect it possesses.[6,9–12] The negative impact on glycemic control that the TCAs seem to possess has not been fully explained at this time.[9] The wise course of action to take if it is decided to initiate TCA treatment in a diabetic patient for any reason will be to acquire baseline clinical and laboratory parameters and to follow the patient closely for changes in these parameters, and if necessary, adjust the dosing of the hypoglycemic treatment or reconsider the use of the TCA treatment.

The efficacy of the TCA is well established concerning the ability to treat painful diabetic neuropathy, and this class of psychotropics is still used today for this purpose, in some cases, even more than the class' use for depression.[4,5,13] The efficacy of the TCAs in treating neuropathic pain appears to be superior to that of the selective serotonin reuptake inhibitors (SSRIs).[4] This has supported the theory that the combination of both the serotonin and norepinephrine components of the TCA are important mechanisms to address this painful syndrome, and thus their possible advantage over the SSRIs regarding this specific issue. With the growing use and proven efficacy of venlafaxine and duloxetine for diabetic neuropathy, perhaps the use of the TCAs for this specific condition may also diminish.[5,9,14–17]

Monoamine oxidase inhibitors

The monoamine oxidase inhibitors (MAOIs) have been available for the treatment of depression for approximately 50 years, but the use of this subclass of antidepressants has been reduced to near zero compared with the newer and safer antidepressant subclasses. It is of special note, however, that the latest Food and Drug Administration (FDA)-approved antidepressant is the MAOI selegiline, which is now available in a transdermal delivery system. This product's new approval for the treatment of depression and the formulation change may prompt some practitioners to reconsider MAOI treatment of depression, especially with the expectation for a diminished risk for drug–food and drug–drug interactions with this new formulation. Historically, this subclass of antidepressants, while very effective for depression, is considered difficult to use due to the need for dietary restrictions and the risk for drug–drug interactions. Limited data regarding the impact of MAOIs on glucose metabolism suggest a possible hypoglycemic effect when they have been prescribed to some patients.[18,19]

Long-term risks of MAOI treatment on DM status are unknown. Weight gain has been reported with the older MAOIs; however, it is not considered a common adverse effect with selegiline. Selegiline has not been adequately studied in patients with DM to make a recommendation for its use in this unique population at this time and, thus, caution and vigilance is warranted with this MAOI if it is prescribed for persons with both DM and depression.

Selective serotonin reuptake inhibitors

The antidepressant subclass of SSRIs has been the most commonly prescribed group of antidepressants for over 10 years. These antidepressants have largely replaced the older TCAs and MAOIs because of their improved safety and toxicity profiles. There are currently six SSRIs available for prescription: fluoxetine, sertraline, paroxetine, fluvoxamine, citalopram, and escitalopram. Some research has been conducted with the use of SSRIs in depressed patients with DM. With respect to fluoxetine and sertraline, some improvement in glucose management may occur along with the expected reduction in depressive symptoms that occurred in both the open-label study with sertraline and the double-blind, placebo-controlled study testing fluoxetine.[2,3] In early studies, weight reduction appeared to be a benefit of SSRIs over the older TCAs. In a review discussing antidepressant treatment options in the diabetic patient by Goodnick, the laboratory and clinical data suggest the benefit of the SSRI class in treating patients with DM.[9] Some of the data for this position are based on studies of fluoxetine for weight loss in both non-diabetic and diabetic obese patients who did not have comorbid depression and most of the studies are of short duration. More recent reports reveal that long-term exposure to SSRIs may also cause a weight gain in some patients.[20] So, whereas an initial and seemingly beneficial weight loss, and possible improvement in glucose parameters such as fasting plasma glucose and HbA_{1c} may occur in some patients receiving SSRI treatment, the clinician should continue monitoring the patient's weight and laboratory results for a possible return to baseline, or even an increase in weight above pretreatment baseline status. There have been reports of improved insulin sensitivity with fluoxetine and even hypoglycemia with sertraline.[21,22] This supports the recommendation for baseline and follow-up monitoring of the diabetic patient receiving SSRIs due to potential changes in laboratory results and possible need for a dosage adjustment of the patient's diabetic treatment regimen.

Serotonin–norepinephrine reuptake inhibitors

The SNRI group of antidepressants is currently composed of venlafaxine and duloxetine. As stated above, the older TCAs could technically qualify for this designation, but are not generally included in this subclass of antidepressants to assist in distinguishing the adverse effect and safety profile of these two newer antidepressants from the TCAs. Neither venlafaxine nor duloxetine has been adequately studied for the treatment of depression in the diabetic population; however, both agents have been studied for the treatment of painful diabetic neuropathy and appear to be efficacious for this painful syndrome in either depressed or non-depressed patients.[14–17] Duloxetine is even FDA-approved for diabetic neuropathy. Interestingly, one psychotropic that is FDA-approved for the treatment of obesity, and not depression, is also a very potent SNRI. And though originally studied as a potential antidepressant, it was eventually developed as a weight loss agent. This agent is sibutramine.[23] Very little recent data support its use as an antidepressant and no data support its use in depressed diabetic patients. However, the mechanisms of action of this agent and its side-effect profile may be a factor in the practitioner's selection of treatment in this population. The risk of increased blood pressure and heart rate is possible with venlafaxine, duloxetine, and sibutramine, largely due to the NE reuptake-inhibiting quality of these agents. The TCAs never really had this side-effect risk because of their α-1 receptor antagonistic effect, essentially providing them with a built-in antihypertensive action which is so significant as to cause orthostasis with the TCA subclass of antidepressants. Orthostasis is not considered a risk with the newer SNRIs. Therefore the noradrenergic effect of the SNRIs on the heart and blood vessels is unopposed, and thus the potential to cause the related side effects of increased heart rate and blood pressure. The TCAs can cause tachycardia, but this is generally due to anticholinergic and orthostatic effects. In studies assessing diabetes laboratory parameters in patients prescribed duloxetine and venlafaxine for diabetic neuropathy, neither agent appeared to worsen the common parameters of glucose, HbA_{1c}, lipids, or even weight, and these agents may potentially improve these important factors in diabetes management.[14–17]

Other antidepressants

Bupropion is unique in the class of antidepressants by being a weak reuptake inhibitor of both dopamine and NE.[6] It is also FDA-approved for smoking cessation, a lifestyle behavior of some patients with DM which may worsen the overall clinical outcome for this patient population. Bupropion has not been adequately studied in the comorbid depressed and diabetic population to make a recommendation for its use over other agents; however, this agent is associated with minimal to no weight gain and occasionally weight loss. There are no negative reports of long-term weight gain or worsening of diabetes laboratory parameters.[24] In a small study assessing the effect of bupropion on sexual functioning in non-depressed diabetic men, there was no negative impact on diabetic control reported and the medication was well tolerated in this subject group.[25] Bupropion may therefore be a viable and effective alternative to consider for the depressed patient with DM, although more research is needed with the use of this agent in this specific population.

Nefazodone and trazodone are antidepressants with 5-HT receptor antagonism and weak reuptake inhibition of 5-HT.[6] Neither antidepressant has been adequately studied to make a recommendation for first-line use in the depressed patient with comorbid diabetes mellitus. Nefazodone is not commonly prescribed today due to the black box warning issued regarding the risk for hepatotoxicity; the branded version of the drug was voluntarily removed from the market, though a generic version of the drug is still available for prescription. There have not been studies assessing this agent's applicability in treating patients with DM and depression; however, a case has been published reporting its potential to cause a hypoglycemic reaction.[26] Trazodone is also rarely prescribed today to treat depression, though it is commonly prescribed at low doses as adjunctive treatment for insomnia. The antihistamine properties of trazodone that contribute to its sedating effects would suggest that weight gain may also be an issue with this agent, though it is not commonly associated with significant weight gain. This drug is rarely used at the appropriately higher doses to treat depression and its use for the treatment of depression with comorbid DM remains untested. One possible explanation for the low risk for weight gain observed with trazodone and nefazodone may be related to their active metabolite, *m*-chlorophenylpiperazine (m-CPP), a compound known to be a potent serotonin receptor agonist and to reduce food intake in animal models.[27,28]

Mirtazapine is an antidepressant with both 5-HT receptor antagonism and α-2 receptor antagonism, along with significant antihistamine properties. It has been on the market for approximately 10 years. No published reports have been found of its use in treating patients with both DM and depression. The ability of this psychotropic agent to cause weight gain is well recognized and documented.[8,24,29–31] Some of the reports of significant weight gain also include reports of hyperglycemia and, given that this medication has some of the same pharmacologic features as other drugs that have been implicated with negative changes in glucose and weight gain, such as the atypical antipsychotics (serotonin and histamine antagonism), the use of mirtazapine in diabetic patients with depression should be cautioned and perhaps this agent should be considered an alternative, only after other agents with a lower risk of worsening a patient's weight or diabetic control have been tried.

Section summary

Given the high comorbidity between DM and depression, it is expected that a significant number of patients with these two disorders, and possibly with other medical conditions such as hypertension, will receive treatment with antidepressants. Though still not fully assessed and studied, there may be potential drug–drug interactions between antidepressants or the other psychotropic agents, and with hypoglycemic agents. This should always be a consideration for the practitioner. There are some reports of hypoglycemia when diabetes medications have been given concomitantly with antidepressants. These combinations may result in either pharmacodynamic, or pharmacokinetic interactions, and further research is needed in this area. A review of this topic by DeVane and Markowitz offers some recommendations when prescribing psychotropics concomitantly with hypoglycemic agents.[32]

At this time, most of the literature addressing antidepressants and DM, or their impact on glucose and weight, suggests that the SSRIs may be appropriate first choices to treat depression in this group of patients; however, the newer SNRIs and bupropion, though less studied, may also offer benefits such as possible weight neutrality and/or analgesic qualities that may also make these antidepressants good choices for the diabetic patient with depression. Table 10.1 provides a guide to the relative risks of the antidepressants that impact diabetic parameters: it was synthesized from the literature.

Bipolar disorder and mood stabilizers

Bipolar disorder is a mood disorder that has been associated with possible increased risk for obesity and DM. The systematic study of the impact of the mood stabilizers on diabetic parameters in large numbers of patients with comorbid DM and bipolar disorder is sorely lacking. Much of the data assessing the impact on glucose and diabetic parameters for the anticonvulsants which are now approved as mood stabilizers, such as valproic acid and carbamazepine, has been generated from their study in epilepsy. Although lithium has been used for decades in the treatment of bipolar disorder and its effect on weight and glucose has been assessed, research on its effect on diabetic control in patients with both bipolar disorder and DM vs its risk of causing DM is still relatively minimal.

Lithium

Lithium can still be considered the 'gold standard' for the treatment of bipolar disorder; however, its historical use and toxicities have created somewhat of a stigma against this medication, and it is used less today than in past decades. This reduced use of lithium may also be due to the recent approval of some of the atypical antipsychotic agents for the treatment of bipolar disorder, thus giving the practitioner more approved treatment options than before and new marketing pressures to use newer agents vs the less-promoted, yet well-established and efficacious lithium. The possible association and potential risks of lithium with diabetes have been reported in the literature for over 35 years.[33,34] However, the cases and studies reveal a varied effect of lithium on glucose and DM. Weight gain with lithium is possible and may have a

Table 10.1   Psychotropic drug impact on diabetes

Drug	Risk of hyperglycemia	Risk of hypoglycemia	Weight change	Comments
Antidepressants				
TCAs	-/+	-/+	↑	↓ neuropathy
MAOIs	-	+	-/↑	
SSRIs				
short-term:	-	+	-/↓	
long-term:	?	-	-/↑	
Venlafaxine	-	-	-	↓ neuropathy
Duloxetine	-	-	-	↓ neuropathy
Bupropion	-	-	-/↓	
Trazodone	+	-	↑	
Nefazodone	-/+	-/+	-/↓	
Mirtazapine	+	-	↑↑	
Mood stabilizers				
Lithium	-/+	-	↑	
Valproic acid	++	-	↑↑	
Carbamazepine	-/+	-	-/↑	↓ neuropathy
Lamotrigine	+	-	-/↑	↓ neuropathy
Antipsychotics				
Phenothiazines	++	-	↑↑	
Haloperidol	+	-	-/↑	
Loxapine	+	-	-/↑	
Molindone	?	-	-/↓	
Thiothixene	?	-	↑	
Atypical agents				*Risk for ↑ lipids*
Clozapine	+++	-	↑↑↑	↑↑
Risperidone	+	-	↑↑	-/↑
Olanzapine	+++	-	↑↑↑	↑↑
Quetiapine	++	-	↑↑	-/↑
Ziprasidone	-/+	-	↑	(-)
Aripiprazole	-/+	-	↑	(-)
Anxiolytics/hypnotics				
Benzodiazepines (BZDs)	-	-/+	-	
'Non-BZDs' (zolpidem, zaleplon, eszopiclone)	?	?	-	
Ramelteon	?	?	?	
Buspirone	-	-/+	-	

- = no significant change expected; + = mild effect on glucose is possible; ++ = moderate effect on glucose is possible (may impair diabetic control and require dose adjustment of hypoglycemic treatment); +++ = significant increase possible (may significantly impair diabetic control and require adjustment of hypoglycemic treatment and limit the use of this medication in some patients with diabetes); ↑ = increase; ↓ = decrease.

negative secondary impact on DM.[35] The mixed literature on lithium and glucose control or its impact upon diabetic status at least warrants baseline assessment and regular follow-up of the patient's diabetic parameters, including weight and renal function.[33-38] Though lithium is associated with the development of drug-induced nephrogenic diabetes insipidus, this side effect has not been associated with the development or specific worsening of DM. Nevertheless, increased clinical and laboratory monitoring is recommended. If a negative impact upon a specific patient's diabetic status is discovered, then the risks and benefits of the lithium treatment, or any mood stabilizer treatment, must be considered if the patient is also experiencing a significant improvement and control in their mood disorder. Thus, continued treatment with lithium may be warranted and more aggressive weight or diabetic management will be necessary through both pharmacologic and non-pharmacologic means.

Valproic acid/sodium valproate

Whereas much discussion and published literature has recently occurred regarding the potential weight gain and impact on DM with the antidepressants and antipsychotic agents, the relationship between valproic acid (VPA) and insulin resistance, weight gain, obesity and other diabetes risk factors has been documented for many years.[39-42] The value of VPA as a mood-stabilizing agent, like lithium, is without question for the long-term management of bipolar disorder. And the possible need for combination pharmacotherapy for some patients with bipolar disorder who may be resistant to monotherapy, and thus require an antipsychotic agent or second mood stabilizer in addition to VPA, may confer a synergistic and increased risk for worsening a patient's comorbid diabetic status. Research regarding VPA and its impact on glucose or insulin sensitivity exists mostly in the treatment of patients receiving VPA for epilepsy, but at this time these data should still be considered valid when extrapolating to the treatment of bipolar disorder until significantly more research and data are generated in the use of VPA in diabetic patients with bipolar disorder. The insulin resistance observed with valproic acid may have more to do with the weight gain and possible obesity than a particular endocrine marker or factor. In addition, the mechanisms of the weight gain associated with VPA have not been fully established. Nevertheless, caution and monitoring should be part of the use of VPA treatment for bipolar disorder or any disorder where the clinician feels VPA would be a useful treatment alternative, especially in patients with comorbid DM.

Carbamazepine

The use of carbamazepine (CBZ) as an alternative for the treatment of bipolar disorder has been a common practice for many years; however, the medication only recently received the FDA approval for the treatment of this disorder as the extended-release product formulation Equetro™. Aside from the data available concerning the use of carbamazepine in treating peripheral diabetic neuropathy, there is little data regarding its applicability in diabetic patients with bipolar disorder. In a study assessing the impact of both VPA and CBZ on endocrine markers in female subjects with epilepsy, the investigators reported an increase in insulin levels with CBZ compared with controls.[41] Case reports and some epilepsy studies also reveal a possible weight gain with CBZ.[43] However, other studies suggest a minimal effect of CBZ on weight in patients with affective or psychotic illness.[44,45] The use of CBZ for the management of chronic pain syndromes such as painful diabetic neuropathy is established and has been common practice for many years.[5,46,47] If further research finds that CBZ has minimal negative effects on diabetes treatment parameters while demonstrating the ability to treat bipolar disorder, then perhaps this would be a viable alternative agent for this group of patients, especially if a comorbid pain syndrome is also present.

Lamotrigine

This anticonvulsant, now approved for relapse prevention and maintenance treatment of bipolar disorder, has not been adequately studied in patients with DM. However, lamotrigine has also not been associated with significant weight gain or worsening of DM and may actually have an additional benefit of reducing painful diabetic neuropathy.[47,48] In a recent retrospective study by Sachs and colleagues, the impact on body weight of lamotrigine was compared with placebo and lithium during maintenance treatment for a year and lamotrigine was found to not increase body weight during this period of treatment, whereas lithium did increase weight during the same time frame.[49] The possible weight neutrality and lack of reports regarding any worsening of DM from lamotrigine compared with other mood stabilizers and antipsychotics suggest that this agent may be an attractive alternative in addressing bipolar disorder in patients with comorbid DM; however, research is needed to fully assess the impact of lamotrigine in this specific population and its use should still be closely monitored until more data are generated. Discussion regarding unapproved agents that are occasionally tried as mood stabilizers, such as topiramate and oxcarbazepine, was intentionally avoided given the minimal data for efficacy and effect on diabetes status at this time. However, these agents may eventually prove to be useful for treating patients with comorbid DM and bipolar disorder.

Antipsychotics

The antipsychotics have historically been used for the acute management of mania. The established efficacy of the older, 'conventional', agents, from chlorpromazine through to haloperidol, still makes the older antipsychotic a possible alternative when choosing an acute treatment for mania. The long-term use of the older, first-generation antipsychotics (FGAs) for the management of bipolar disorder is not as well studied, and the longer the exposure of patients to older antipsychotics, the greater the possible risk for the development of the irreversible movement disorder, tardive dyskinesia. Today, it is established that the 'atypical' antipsychotics, also referred to as second-generation antipsychotics (SGAs), are effective for the acute management of bipolar disorder and may possibly be considered for longer-term management of the disorder in select patients. There has been a surge in SGA prescribing for bipolar disorder, partly because all of the medications (except clozapine) have received FDA approval for the indication and thus are being extensively marketed, with research literature that supports their use. With an apparent increased risk for individuals with bipolar disorder to develop DM independent of their pharmacologic treatment modality and the potential risk of exacerbation of DM with an SGA, a significant level of monitoring should be implemented with the use of these agents to manage bipolar disorder, especially in patients with pre-existing DM. A longer discussion regarding the SGAs and their risk for hyperglycemia and worsening diabetic parameters appears later in this chapter under a section on the treatment of schizophrenia with these agents, since little research has thus far focused on SGAs and long-term risk for glucose and metabolic abnormalities in patients with bipolar disorder and comorbid DM.

Section summary

With the reporting of an increased risk of DM in persons with bipolar disorder, and the potential for many of the agents used to treat bipolar disorder to affect glucose, insulin, lipids, and weight, increased monitoring is recommended in patients with these co-occurring conditions. Given that drug-related adverse effects, such as weight gain, also significantly and negatively affect adherence with medication treatment for bipolar disorder and may lead to an exacerbation of diabetic status, every effort should be made to assess and encourage adherence to the complete treatment regimen. Ongoing education and behavioral, exercise, and nutritional counseling should also be a part of a patient's treatment regimen to minimize the potential negative impact of medication-related adverse effects on the patient's treatment and their perceptions and expectations of the treatment.

Schizophrenia

The increased risk and prevalence of DM in patients with schizophrenia is addressed in Chapter 2, with possible explanations related to genetic predisposition, lifestyle, and eating behaviors. The incidence and prevalence of diabetes in this population is further complicated by the large majority of patients with schizophrenia who are chronically treated with antipsychotic medications, thus complicating the assessment of the cause for this increased prevalence. The likely explanation is that a multifactorial impact exists. Given that the antipsychotics are the mainstay of treatment for the individual with schizophrenia and that a significant number of these persons will develop, or already have developed, DM during the course of their treatment, then a discussion of the impact of antipsychotics on diabetic parameters is necessary.

Antipsychotics

A considerable amount of research and literature has been generated in the last 10 years regarding the antipsychotics, with most attention being paid to the atypical antipsychotics: clozapine, risperidone, olanzapine, quetiapine, ziprasidone and aripiprazole. They are also referred to as SGAs and are commonly compared against the FGAs such as chlorpromazine, perphenazine, fluphenazine, and haloperidol, which are considered as the popular representatives of this older group of agents. Pharmacologically, the SGAs usually, but not always, have a greater affinity for the 5HT-2 receptors than the FGAs, compared with their binding affinity for the DA-2 receptor, and this difference in receptor affinities is believed to contribute to their 'atypicality'.[50,51] The FGAs are still considered effective for the treatment of the positive symptoms (delusions, hallucinations, agitation) of schizophrenia and recent evidence has reinforced the potential effectiveness of perphenazine, as being comparable to the effectiveness of some newer SGAs such as risperidone, olanzapine, quetiapine, and ziprasidone.[52] However, the beneficial effect of FGAs on negative symptoms associated with many clinical presentations of schizophrenia is limited, with the FGAs having the potential to even worsen or induce aspects of negative symptoms or affective symptoms. This therapeutic limitation, along with the continued and relatively high risk of adverse extrapyramidal symptoms (EPS) such as dystonia, akathisia, and pseudoparkinsonism, and even the generally irreversible movement disorder of tardive dyskinesia, have made these agents second-line therapies today. However, the literature strongly reports the risk for weight gain, hyperglycemia, and possible insulin resistance with the SGAs, even more so than with the FGAs. And there also appear to be different levels of risk for hyperglycemia and weight gain among the six current agents in this SGA class. The mechanisms of antipsychotic-induced hyperglycemia and insulin resistance are not completely understood, but may not be related to an agent's ability to cause weight gain. Possible mechanisms explaining the reason for weight gain with antipsychotics include the antihistamine and antiserotonin properties of some of these agents affecting energy homeostasis, glucose transporter dysregulation, psychomotor activity, appetite, and satiety.[28,53–56]

First-generation antipsychotics

The acute and long-term uses of the older FGAs for the management of psychotic illness are well studied and established. Newly developed antipsychotics are still commonly compared with the older FGAs such as haloperidol for efficacy and tolerability before approval for general use on the US market. This further reinforces the current FGAs as efficacious for the treatment of psychosis. The risk of hyperglycemia with the use of chlorpromazine was reported many years ago and these reports are generally consistent, though usually after short periods of observation.[57-59] Weight gain has also been reported with many of the FGAs.[60,61] Interestingly, even after being available and used for over 20 years, some FGAs have minimal to no reports of hyperglycemia or weight gain associated with their use. With the potential minimal impact on weight and diabetic parameters of some of the older FGAs such as haloperidol and molindone, or the limited reporting of hyperglycemia with other non-phenothiazine agents, the FGAs should not be dismissed as viable treatment alternatives for patients with comorbid DM and psychotic illness. However, the higher risk of both reversible and irreversible EPS with the FGAs will probably continue to limit their use in current practice.

Second-generation antipsychotics

The atypical antipsychotics or SGAs are now considered to be first-line agents for the treatment of psychotic illness. Their lower risk for EPS, along with their potential advantages over the FGAs in certain aspects of schizophrenia, such as greater improvement in negative, affective, and cognitive symptoms, has reinforced their place as first-line treatment alternatives with the exception of clozapine use, which is limited for other reasons such as the adverse effects of agranulocytosis and seizures. However, the continued observations and publications of the negative impact of SGAs on weight and glycemic control may significantly limit their use in treating patients with comorbid DM and schizophrenia. This increased risk for hyperglycemia, possibly resulting in diabetic ketoacidosis, coma, and death, even in the presence of no associated weight gain, has prompted the FDA to require that all of the SGAs include a warning regarding an increased risk for hyperglycemia in the product labeling of these agents. At the time the warning was issued by the FDA, there was very little evidence of hyperglycemia or drug-induced diabetes secondary to ziprasidone or aripiprazole; however, these agents are relatively new to the market and are the least-prescribed agents in the SGA class at this time, which may account for the low number of cases reported.[62] This appropriately conservative position by the FDA on this issue should prompt all prescribers of antipsychotics to exercise caution with the use of these agents in patients with preexisting diabetes mellitus. A joint conference of the American Diabetic Association, the American Psychiatric Association, the American Association of Clinical Endocrinologists, and the North American Association for the Study of Obesity was held to address the growing issue of SGA-related hyperglycemia, weight gain, lipid changes, and risk for diabetes. As a result of the conference, guidelines for the use and monitoring of the SGAs were developed.[63] The relative risks of the SGAs on affecting weight, glucose, and lipids reported by this conference have been incorporated into Table 10.1.

The risk of hyperglycemia appears to be greatest with clozapine and olanzapine, with a lesser risk related to risperidone and quetiapine.[53,63–68] A series of papers from Koller and colleagues have assessed the published and FDA-submitted case reports regarding the older SGAs and their relationship to hyperglycemia and DM.[69–72] At this time, ziprasidone and aripiprazole appear to demonstrate the lowest risk for causing hyperglycemia or DM, though admittedly, these newer agents have also been the least prescribed and their true risk may not be fully determined at this time. The risks for causing increases in weight have been associated with all of the SGAs, and again, the highest risk for weight gain appears to be associated with the use of clozapine and olanzapine, with the lowest risks associated, at this time, with ziprasidone and aripiprazole.[61,63,73]

No matter which SGA is being considered and prescribed, the recommendations for monitoring non-diabetic patients receiving one of these agents are for the baseline and pretreatment assessment of personal and family history of obesity, diabetes, dyslipidemia, hypertension, or cardiovascular disease; the patient's height and weight for body mass index determination; waist circumference; blood pressure; fasting plasma glucose; and fasting lipid profile.[63] The recommendations for follow-up monitoring suggest assessment of weight monthly for 3 months, then quarterly. If a >5% weight gain from baseline occurs, then switching to another antipsychotic should be considered. Fasting glucose, lipid profile, and blood pressure were recommended to be reassessed at 3 months and annually thereafter, with lipids recommended to be reassessed every 5 years unless otherwise indicated. These recommendations were made for all patients receiving SGAs and not specifically for patients with pre-existing DM. The guidelines recommend more frequent monitoring in those patients at higher risk for developing DM, but this is left to the discretion of the clinician. Given that this chapter is meant to address the management of patients with existing DM with comorbid psychiatric illness and the risk of these agents to cause diabetes or exacerbate certain diabetic parameters, it is the recommendation of this author for a *much more frequent level of monitoring* of fasting glucose, HbA$_{1c}$, lipid profile, weight, and other diabetic parameters. Some cases of changes in glucose secondary to SGAs report a relatively rapid increase in glucose and lipids within days to weeks of initiation of antipsychotic treatment, even without associated weight gain, and therefore it may be necessary to monitor these parameters monthly for the first 3–6 months and semiannually thereafter.[69,70] If any clinical or laboratory measurements indicate a worsening of the patient's diabetes status, then more frequent assessment is recommended and reconsideration of the SGA selection should be taken into account and compared with the level of the patient's clinical response to the antipsychotic in treating the mental illness.

Section summary

Despite the risks for possible worsening of diabetic control with the antipsychotics, their effectiveness in managing psychotic illness warrants their use in this population. Aggressive and ongoing lifestyle management to address behaviors such as decreased physical activity, smoking, and eating habits, all of which can worsen the control of diabetes, along with the continued management of other comorbid disorders such as hypertension and dyslipidemia, are necessary. Given the relatively poor insight and sometimes poor motivation and life skills of individuals with schizophrenia to manage their own diabetes through non-pharmacologic and pharmacologic means, the overall outcome of this unique population can be poor if not properly supervised by health care professionals. In patients with established DM, serious consideration should be given to select antipsychotic agents with minimal risks of exacerbating the patient's diabetic status, and frequent monitoring of diabetic parameters is warranted.

Anxiety and anxiolytics

Very little published clinical data exist regarding the pharmacologic management of patients with anxiety disorders and comorbid DM. Non-pharmacologic interventions, such as cognitive behavioral therapy, should be considered in this group of patients given the relative success of this intervention and the potential avoidance of risk of exacerbating the patient's diabetes with a medication. Though the reduction in stress-related cortisol activity may provide a beneficial effect on insulin release and glucose control, the impact of anxiolytics on this system are mixed. The antidepressant–anxiolytics, such as the SSRIs, have been discussed earlier in this chapter and their impact on weight and other possible diabetic parameters would probably apply to the anxiety disorders but these agents have not been systematically studied in diabetic patients with anxiety disorders. However, the same advantages and disadvantages discussed earlier in this chapter with antidepressants should be considered in the anxiety disorders until more data is generated.

Benzodiazepines

Small in-vivo and in-vitro studies have suggested the possibility of impaired glucose metabolism or insulin release with benzodiazepines, though given the widespread use of benzodiazepines over the past four decades, if this possible negative impact was meaningful, then significantly more case reports and studies would have been generated by now. Nevertheless, the use of the benzodiazepines may affect diabetic parameters.[74–77] Most of the published data are reporting short-term trials and some of these trials also report improvement in diabetic parameters such as glucose levels.[74] Sufficient long-term data are not available for assessment and therefore the limited time frames and small numbers of subjects in these cases or trials make it difficult to recommend a particular agent or specific monitoring in anxious patients receiving benzodiazepines at this time.

Other anxiolytics: hydroxyzine, antipsychotics, and buspirone

The impact of hydroxyzine on glucose control and DM is unknown. The use of the older antipsychotics for the treatment of symptoms of anxiety has been largely replaced by the newer antidepressant–anxiolytics and the emerging use of atypical SGAs for severe anxiety disorders such as post-traumatic stress disorder or resistant obsessive compulsive disorder. If patients with a severe and refractory anxiety disorder and comorbid DM are being considered for treatment with an

SGA, then the prior cautions and recommendations for increased monitoring of these patients should still be at the forefront of the clinician's treatment plan. The effect of buspirone on diabetic parameters is believed at this time to be either neutral or positive, based on limited animal research.[78,79] Human studies are not available for a full assessment regarding the place of buspirone in treating diabetic and anxious patients. However, the lack of any case reports after being on the market and available for over 15 years is encouraging for buspirone's usefulness in this specific population.

Insomnia

A large number of patients with either DM or psychiatric illness will have the complaint of insomnia and many may be prescribed hypnotic agents to address their insomnia. The impact of hypnotic agents in patients with comorbid DM has not been adequately assessed and therefore no recommendations other than caution can be made at this time. In one small and short-term study assessing an imidazopyridine, similar to zolpidem, the investigators suggest that an imidazopyridine derivative may inhibit glucose-induced insulin secretion.[80] One study assessing cardiovascular parameters and nocturnal blood pressure changes in diabetic patients given zolpidem did not report any negative impact on diabetic or cardiovascular status as a result of zolpidem administration.[81] Data regarding zaleplon and eszopiclone are not available.

The benzodiazepines available for use in the short-term management of insomnia have not been adequately studied in patients with DM to make recommendations for their use in this population. The antihistamines and low-dose trazodone or TCAs have also not been adequately studied for their impact on DM and comorbid insomnia; however, their potential benefit for patients with diabetic neuropathy and insomnia may warrant their consideration for use in that subpopulation of patients, as long as diabetes status is continually monitored. Given the potential worsening of weight and diabetes control with medications such as mirtazapine and quetiapine, which have been used clinically for insomnia, though with little evidence-based support, the use of these two agents in diabetic patients with insomnia is not recommended by this author. There are also no reported data on the impact of the newest approved hypnotic agent ramelteon, a melatonin receptor agonist, and therefore use of this agent in the diabetic population with insomnia warrants caution at this time.

Conclusions

The use of psychotropics in patients with psychiatric illness and comorbid DM is an inevitable occurrence during medical and psychiatric practice, especially in light of the growing prevalence of these conditions. However, research in these specific patient populations who are prescribed psychotropics is generally lacking and though the research literature has recently reported data regarding the potential negative impact of the older SGAs, such as olanzapine and clozapine, the full impact of the newer SGAs, ziprasidone and aripiprazole, remains to be seen. The various antidepressants may have a mixed effect on diabetes control and their use also warrants close monitoring of diabetic parameters. Certain mood stabilizers, such as valproic acid, may have a greater negative impact on diabetes control compared with newer agents such as lamotrigine; however, further research is needed in the area of mood stabilizers and diabetes management. Therefore caution should be exercised when prescribing any psychotropic for the patient with DM. When possible, non-pharmacologic interventions should be implemented along with significant education and counseling regarding lifestyle behaviors, diet, and exercise, along with medication adherence with all pharmacologic treatments for both psychiatric and diabetes management to ensure optimal outcomes for this complicated patient population.

References

1. Lustman PJ, Griffith LS, Clouse RE et al. Effects of nortriptyline on depression and glycemic control in diabetes: results of a double-blind, placebo-controlled trial. Psychosom Med 1997; 59: 241–50.
2. Goodnick PJ, Kumar AH, Henry JH et al. Sertraline in coexisting major depression and diabetes mellitus. Psychopharmacol Bull 1997; 33: 261–4.
3. Lustman PJ, Freedland KE, Griffith LS et al. Fluoxetine for depression in diabetes: a randomized, double-blind, placebo-controlled trial. Diabetes Care 2000; 23: 618–25.
4. Max MB, Lynch SA, Muir J et al. Effects of desipramine, amitriptyline, and fluoxetine in diabetic neuropathy. N Engl J Med 1992; 326: 1250–6.

5. Sindrup SH, Jensen TS. Efficacy of pharmacological treatments of neuropathic pain: an update and effect related to mechanism of drug action. Pain 1999; 83: 389–400.

6. Richelson E. Pharmacology of antidepressants. Mayo Clin Proc 2001; 76: 511–27.

7. Cole JO, Bodkin JA. Antidepressant drug side effects. J Clin Psychiatry 1990; 51(Suppl 2): 21–6.

8. Fava M. Weight gain and antidepressants. J Clin Psychiatry 2000; 62(Suppl 23): 13–22.

9. Goodnick PJ. Use of antidepressants in treatment of comorbid diabetes mellitus and depression as well as in diabetic neuropathy. Ann Clin Psychiatry 2001; 13: 31–41.

10. Katz LM, Fochtmann LF, Pato MT. Clomipramine, fluoxetine, and glucose control. Ann Clin Psychiatry 1991; 3: 271–4.

11. Kaplan JM, Mass JW, Pixley JM et al. Use of imipramine in diabetics. JAMA 1960; 174: 511–17.

12. True BL, Perry PJ, Burns EA. Profound hypoglycemia with the addition of a tricyclic antidepressant to maintenance sulfonylurea therapy. Am J Psychiatry 1987; 144: 1220–21.

13. Sindrup SH, Gram LF, Skjold T et al. Clomipramine vs desipramine vs placebo in the treatment of diabetic neuropathy symptoms. A double-blind cross-over study. Br J Clin Pharmacol 1990; 30: 683–91.

14. Kaminski-Price C, Rey JA, Cruz W et al. Venlafaxine for the treatment of painful diabetic neuropathy. Presented at the International Association for the Study of Pain (IASP) 9th World Congress on Pain, Vienna, Austria, August 1999.

15. Kunz NR, Goli V, Entsuah R et al. Diabetic neuropathic pain management with venlafaxine extended release. Eur Neuro Psychopharmacol 2000; 10(Suppl 3): S389.

16. Goldstein DJ, Lu Y, Detke MJ et al. Duloxetine vs placebo in patients with painful diabetic neuropathy. Pain 2005; 116: 109–18.

17. Raskin J, Smith TR, Wong K et al. Duloxetine versus routine care in the long-term management of diabetic peripheral neuropathic pain. J Palliat Med 2006; 9: 29–40.

18. Cooper AJ, Ashcroft G. Potentiation of insulin hypoglycemia by MAOI antidepressant drugs. Lancet 1966; 1: 407–9.

19. Adnitt PI. Hypoglycemic action of monoamine oxidase inhibitors (MAOI's). Diabetes 1968; 17: 628–33.

20. Sussman N, Ginsberg D. Weight gain associated with SSRI's. Prim Psychiatry 1998; 5: 28–37.

21. Maheux P, Ducros F, Bourque J et al. Fluoxetine improves insulin sensitivity in obese patients with non-insulin-dependent diabetes mellitus independently of weight loss. Int J Obesity 1997; 21: 97–102.

22. Pollak PT, Mukherjee SD, Fraser AD. Sertraline-induced hypoglycemia. Ann Pharmacother 2001; 35: 1371–4.

23. Luque CA, Rey JA. Sibutramine: a serotonin-norepinephrine reuptake inhibitor for the treatment of obesity. Ann Pharmacother 1999; 33: 968–78.

24. Masand PS, Gupta S. Long-term side effects of newer-generation antidepressants: SSRIs, venlafaxine, nefazodone, bupropion, and mirtazapine. Ann Clin Psychiatry 2002; 14: 175–82.

25. Rowland DL, Myers L, Culver A et al. Bupropion and sexual function: a placebo-controlled prospective study on diabetic men with erectile dysfunction. J Clin Psychopharmacol 1997; 17: 350–7.

26. Warnock JK. Nefazodone-induced hypoglycemia. Am J Psychiatry 1997; 154: 288–9.

27. Walsh AES, Smith KA, Oldman AD et al. m-Chlorophenylpiperazine decreases food intake in a test meal. Psychopharmacology 1994; 116: 120–2.

28. Tecott LH, Sun LM, Akana SF et al. Eating disorder and epilepsy in mice lacking 5-HT-2C serotonin receptors. Nature 1995; 374: 542–6.

29. Fawcett J, Barkin RL. Review of the results from clinical studies on the efficacy, safety and tolerability of mirtazapine for the treatment of patients with major depression. J Affect Disord 1998; 51: 267–85.

30. Fisfalen ME, Hsiung RC. Glucose dysregulation and mirtazapine-induced weight gain. Am J Psychiatry 2001; 160: 797.

31. Laimer M, Kramer-Reinstadler K, Rauchenzauner M et al. Effect of mirtazapine treatment on body composition and metabolism. J Clin Psychiatry 2006; 67: 421–4.

32. DeVane CL, Markowitz JS. Psychoactive drug interactions with pharmacotherapy for diabetes. Psychopharmacol Bull 2002; 36: 40–52.

33. Van der Velde CD, Gordon MW. Manic-depressive illness, diabetes mellitus, and lithium carbonate. Arch Gen Psychiatry 1969; 21: 478–85.

34. Lazarus JH. Endocrine and Metabolic Effects of Lithium. New York: Plenum Medical Book Co, 1986.

35. Garland EJ, Remick RA, Zis AP. Weight gain: a side-effect with antidepressants and lithium. J Clin Psychopharmacol 1988; 8: 323–30.

36. Muller-Oerlinghausen B, Passoth PM, Poser W et al. Impaired glucose tolerance in long-term lithium-treated patients. Int Pharmacopsychiatry 1979; 14: 350–62.

37. Jones GR, Lazarus JH, Davies CJ, Greenwood RH. The effect of short term lithium carbonate in Type II diabetes mellitus. Horm Metab Res 1983; 15: 422–4.

38. Vestergaard P, Schou M. Does long-term lithium treatment induce diabetes mellitus? Neuropsychobiology 1987; 17: 130–2.

39. Dinesen H, Gram L, Anderson C, Dam M. Weight gain during treatment with valproate. Acta Neurol Scand 1984; 69: 65–9.

40. Breum L, Astrup A, Gram L. Metabolic changes during treatment with valproate in humans: implication for untoward weight gain. Metabolism 1992; 41: 666–70.

41. Isojarvi JIT, Laatikainen TJ, Knip M et al. Obesity and endocrine disorders in women taking valproate for epilepsy. Ann Neurol 1996; 39: 579–84.

42. Verrotti A, Basciani F, De Simone M et al. Insulin resistance in epileptic girls who gain weight after therapy with valproic acid. J Child Neurol 2002; 17: 265–8.

43. Lampl Y, Eshel Y, Rapaport A et al. Weight gain, increased appetite, and excessive food intake induced by carbamazepine. Clin Neuropharmacol 1991; 14: 251–5.

44. Joffe RT, Post RM, Uhde TW. Effect of carbamazepine on body weight in affectively ill patients. J Clin Psychiatry 1986; 47: 313–4.

45. Vieweg V, Godleski L, Hundley P et al. Antipsychotic drugs, lithium, carbamazepine, and abnormal diurnal weight gain in psychosis. Neuropsychopharmacology 1989; 2: 39–43.

46. Rull JA, Quibrera R, Gonzalez-Millan H et al. Symptomatic treatment of peripheral diabetic neuropathy with carbamazepine (Tegretol): double blind crossover trial. Diabetologia 1969; 5: 215–18.

47. Jensen TS. Anticonvulsants in neuropathic pain: rationale and clinical evidence. Eur J Pain 2002; 6(Suppl A): 61–8.

48. Eisenberg E, Lurie Y, Braker C et al. Lamotrigine reduces painful diabetic neuropathy. Neurology 2001; 57: 505–9.

49. Sachs G, Bowden C, Calabrese JR et al. Effects of lamotrigine and lithium on body weight during maintenance treatment of bipolar 1 disorder. Bipolar Disord 2006; 8: 175–81.

50. Richelson E, Souder T. Binding of antipsychotic drugs to human brain receptors: focus on newer generation compounds. Life Sci 2000; 68: 29–39.

51. Meltzer HY, Matsubara S, Lee JC. The ratios of serotonin2 and dopamine2 affinities differentiate atypical and typical antipsychotic drugs. Psychopharmacol Bull 1989; 25: 390–2.
52. Lieberman JA, Stroup TS, McEoy JP et al. Effectiveness of antipsychotic drugs in patients with chronic schizophrenia. N Engl J Med 2005; 353: 1209–23.
53. Wirshing DA, Boyd JA, Meng LR et al. The effects of novel antipsychotics on glucose and lipid levels. J Clin Psychiatry 2002; 63: 856–65.
54. Reynolds GP, Zhang Z, Zhang X. Polymorphism of the promoter region of the serotonin 5-HT(2C) receptor gene and clozapine-induced weight gain. Am J Psychiatry 2003; 160: 677–9.
55. Heiser P, Singh JS, Krieg JC et al. Effects of different antipsychotics and the antidepressant mirtazapine on glucose transporter mRNA levels in human blood cells. J Psychiatr Res 2006; 40: 374–9.
56. Sakata T, Yoshimatsu H, Kurokawa M. Hypothalamic neuronal histamine: implications of its homeostatic control of energy metabolism. Nutrition 1997; 13: 403–11.
57. Arneson GA. Phenothiazine derivatives and glucose metabolism. J Neuropsychiatr 1964; 5: 181–98.
58. Erle G, Basso M, Federspil G et al. Effect of chlorpromazine on blood glucose and plasma insulin in man. Eur J Clin Pharmacol 1977; 11: 15–18.
59. Pandit MK, Burke J, Gutafson AB et al. Drug-induced disorders of glucose tolerance. Ann Internal Med 1993; 118: 529–39.
60. Doss FW. The effect of antipsychotic drugs on body weight: a retrospective review. J Clin Psychiatry 1979; 40: 528–30.
61. Allison DB, Mentore JL, Heo M et al. Antipsychotic-induced weight gain: a comprehensive research synthesis. Am J Psychiatry 1999; 156: 1686–96.
62. Sanchez-Barranco P. New onset of diabetes mellitus with ziprasidone: a case report. J Clin Psychiatry 2005; 66: 268–9.
63. American Diabetes Association, American Psychiatric Association, American Association of Clinical Endocrinologists, North American Association for the Study of Obesity. Consensus development conference on antipsychotic drugs and obesity and diabetes. Diabetes Care 2004; 27: 596–601.
64. Henderson DC, Cagliero E, Gray C et al. Clozapine, diabetes mellitus, weight gain, and lipid abnormalities: a five-year naturalistic study. Am J Psychiatry 2000; 157: 975–81.
65. Gianfrancesco FD, Grogg AL, Mahmoud RA et al. Differential effects of risperidone, olanzapine, clozapine, and conventional antipsychotics on type 2 diabetes: findings from a large health plan database. J Clin Psychiatry 2002; 63: 920–30.
66. Koro CE, Fedder DO, L'Italien GJ et al. Assessment of independent effect of olanzapine and risperidone on risk of diabetes among patients with schizophrenia: population based nested case-control study. BMJ 2002; 325: 243.
67. Newcomer JW, Haupt DW, Fucetola R et al. Abnormalities in glucose regulation during antipsychotic treatment of schizophrenia. Arch Gen Psychiatry 2002; 59: 337–45.
68. Howes OD, Bhatnager A, Gaughran FP et al. A prospective study of impairment in glucose control caused by clozapine without changes in insulin resistance. Am J Psychiatry 2004; 161: 361–3.
69. Koller EA, Scheider B, Bennett K et al. Clozapine-associated diabetes. Am J Med 2001; 111: 716–23.
70. Koller EA, Doraiswamy PM. Olanzapine-associated diabetes mellitus. Pharmacotherapy 2002; 22: 841–52.

71. Koller EA, Cross JT, Doraiswamy PM et al. Risperidone-associated diabetes mellitus: a pharmacovigilance study. Pharmacotherapy 2003; 23: 735–44.
72. Koller EA, Weber J, Doraiswamy PM et al. A survey of reports of quetiapine-associated hyperglycemia and diabetes mellitus. J Clin Psychiatry 2004; 65: 857–63.
73. Wetterling T. Bodyweight gain with atypical antipsychotics. A comparative review. Drug Saf 2001; 24: 1017–18.
74. Lustman PJ, Griffith LS, Clouse RE et al. Effects of alprazolam on glucose regulation in diabetes: results of a double-blind, placebo controlled trial. Diabetes Care 1995; 18: 1133–9.
75. Gram LF, Christensen L, Kristensen CB et al. Suppression of plasma cortisol after oral administration of oxazepam in man. Br J Clin Pharmacol 1984; 17: 176–8.
76. Okada S, Ichiki K, Tanokuchi S et al. Effect of an anxiolytic on lipid profile in non-insulin-dependent diabetes mellitus. J Int Med Res 1994; 22: 338–42.
77. Zumoff B, Hellman L. Aggravation of diabetic hyperglycemia by chlordiazepoxide. JAMA 1977; 237: 1960–1.
78. Dixit RK, Puri JN, Sharma MK et al. Effect of anxiolytics on blood sugar level in rabbits. Indian J Exp Biol 2001; 39: 378–80.
79. Sugimoto Y, Takashima N, Noma T et al. Effects of the serotonergic anxiolytic buspirone on plasma glucose and glucose-induced hyperglycemia in mice. J Pharmacol Sci 2003; 93: 446–50.
80. Bottai T, Cartault F, Pouget R et al. An imidazopyridine anxiolytic alters glucose tolerance in patients: a pilot investigation. Clin Neuropharmacol 1995; 18: 79–82.
81. Rachmani R, Shenhav G, Slavachevsky I, Levy Z, Ravid M. Use of a mild sedative helps to identify true non-dippers by ABPM: a study in patients with diabetes mellitus and hypertension. Blood Press Monit 2004; 9: 65–9.

Chapter 11

Treatment options for diabetic peripheral neuropathic pain

Maria D Llorente and B Eliot Cole

Introduction

The main goals of treatment for diabetic peripheral neuropathy pain (DPNP) symptoms are primary prevention and symptom management. Prior to initiating care, practitioners and patients should establish end-points for treatment. If practitioners and patients are not in agreement from the outset, frustration, misunderstandings, and false expectations may occur. When pain reduction is the goal, the amount of reduction should be mutually determined and quantifiable: 30%, 50%, or 75% within 1, 2, or 3 months of treatment. If absolute pain elimination is not expected from the treatment, practitioners must clarify this with patients. Failing to communicate the intent of therapy inevitably leads to patient dissatisfaction, inappropriate use of medication, unsanctioned dose escalations, 'doctor-shopping', and other troublesome behaviors. As with other aspects of diabetes mellitus (DM) management, patients must be empowered to 'self-manage' their own care.

Prevention and glycemic control

Since a major pathophysiologic etiology of diabetic peripheral neuropathy (DPN) is thought to be hyperglycemia, tight control of blood glucose is paramount. Several studies have confirmed that maintenance of near-normal glucose levels prevents the development, and slows the progression, of DPN. Improving vascular disease risk factors (control blood pressure, cholesterol, and triglyceride levels) may also be beneficial.

Prevention and diabetic foot care

Patients with DM must be taught to inspect all aspects of their feet (in-between toes, heels, soles, etc.) daily for redness, injury, blisters, or infection. Mirrors may be needed. Any debris, gravel, or similar objects that might cause pressure or irritation found in shoes should be removed. Redness, swelling, or signs of early infection that are detected should immediately be reported to the health care provider.

Feet should be washed daily in lukewarm water and towel dried between toes and around toe nails, which should be carefully trimmed. Shoes should be wide enough in the toes, provide good arch support, and new shoes should only be worn for 1 or 2 hours, followed by careful inspection of the feet for any redness. Until redness resolves and shoes are broken in properly, they must not be worn throughout the day.

Patients with DM should avoid the following: being on their feet without wearing protective shoes; using stockings with tight elastic bands that restrict blood flow; and exposing their feet to hot water, electric blankets, or heating pads.[1] Following these suggestions can substantially lower the risk of ulceration and amputation.

Symptom management and medication trials

In many cases, symptom management will require trials of multiple medications in various combinations (Table 11.1), usually for non-FDA (Food and Drug Administration)-approved indications (off-label use). The use of time limits for response and/or development of toxicity is helpful to assure that benefits (relief of pain) justify incumbent risks. Table 11.1 also includes 'numbers needed to treat' (NNT) information. The NNT is the calculated number of patients a clinician needs to treat with the medication in order for one of those patients to experience more than 50% pain relief. This number can facilitate comparison of treatment efficacy. The smaller the number, the greater the likelihood of relieving pain.

Table 11.1 Non-opioid medications used to treat diabetic neuropathic pain

Medication	Usual dosage (mg/day)	NNT	Possible mechanism of action	Adverse effect considerations
TCAs				
Secondary amines:			Inhibition of NE and 5-HT reuptake; Sodium channel blockade	Contraindicated in 2nd and 3rd degree heart block, prolonged QT intervals, arrhythmias, recent MI, narrow angle glaucoma; should not be used in elderly as first-line treatment; ↑ weight; anticholinergic (use with caution in BPH, constipation); use cautiously in hepatic disease
Desipramine	10–200	2.2		
Nortriptyline	10–150	N/A		
Tertiary amines:				
Imipramine	10–200	N/A		
Amitriptyline	10–150	2.1		
Clomipramine	25–200	N/A		
Newer antidepressants				
Bupropion SR	100–400	N/A	Inhibition of NE and DA reuptake	Can lower seizure threshold
Venlafaxine ER	150–225	4.5	Inhibition of NE and 5-HT reuptake	Nausea, somnolence; use with tramadol can lead to serotonin syndrome
Duloxetine[ab]	60–120	N/A	Inhibition of NE and 5-HT reuptake	Nausea, use with tramadol can lead to serotonin syndrome; anticholinergic; discontinuation syndrome, sexual dysfunction
Anticonvulsants				
Carbamazepine	400–800	3.3	Decreased sodium channel conductance; inhibits ectopic electrical discharges	Anticholinergic, blood dyscrasias, elevated liver function tests, weight gain, drug–drug interactions, SIADH

continued

Table 11.1 Continued

Medication	Usual dosage (mg/day)	NNT	Possible mechanism of action	Adverse effect considerations
Oxcarbazepine	600–1200	N/A	Membrane stabilizer	Weak hepatic induction
Pregabalin[a]	300–600		Calcium channel binder; modulates calcium influx and release of excitatory neurotransmitters	Somnolence, dizziness, peripheral edema, weight gain, dry mouth, nausea
Gabapentin	900–3600	3.8	↑ GABA synthesis, non-NMDA receptor antagonism, calcium channel binder, modulates calcium influx and release of excitatory neurotransmitters	Sedation, dizziness Dosage reduction in renal failure: Cr Cl 30–60: max dose: 600 mg/day Cr Cl 15–30: max dose: 300 mg/day Dialysis: max dose: 200–300 mg after dialysis session
Lamotrigine	200–400	N/A	Sodium channel blockade	Ataxia, incoordination, blurred vision, double vision, rash, Stevens–Johnson syndrome
Topiramate	100–400	N/A	Inhibition of sodium and calcium channel; inhibition of glutamate-mediated excitation	Paresthesia, constipation, dry mouth, gastritis, ↓ weight, difficulty with memory, anorexia, depression mood, blurred vision, eye pain, ocular redness

NNT = numbers needed to treat; TCAs = tricyclic antidepressants; NE = norepinephrine; 5-HT = 5-hydroxytryptamine (serotonin); MI = myocardial infarction; BPH = benign prostatic hypertrophy; SR = sustained release; ER = extended release; D = dopamine; SIADH = syndrome of inappropriate antidiuretic hormone secretion; GABA = γ-aminobutyric acid; NMDA = N-methyl-D-aspartate; Cr Cl = creatinine clearance; DPNP = diabetic peripheral neuropathic pain.

[a]FDA-approved to treat DPNP.
[b]Licensed in UK to treat DPNP.

Antidepressants

Duloxetine, a serotonin and norepinephrine reuptake inhibitor, is the only antidepressant available in the USA approved by the FDA for the treatment of DPNP.[2,3] Duloxetine is associated with discontinuation symptoms, so that it should be gradually tapered. Suicidal ideation has been linked with its use, so that patients started on this medication should be initially screened for suicidal ideas and regularly monitored for onset of these ideations. Patients should also be advised that suicidal ideations may develop and to contact their health care provider immediately if this were to occur.

Tricyclic antidepressants (TCAs) are commonly prescribed for all types of neuropathic pain and have been first-line therapy for more than 30 years.[4–10] There are two classes of TCAs: secondary amines (nortriptyline, desipramine) and tertiary amines (amitriptyline, imipramine, and clomipramine). The secondary amines exhibit fewer anticholinergic side effects and less sedation, but should still be used very cautiously in the elderly, if at all. Their analgesic effects may be due to blockade of sodium channels, but could also be related to inhibition of both norepinephrine and serotonin reuptake. The analgesic effects are, however, independent of any antidepressant effect.[5] Dosages are typically started at the lowest level, and gradually titrated upwards at 10–25 mg/week. In patients with both pain and depression, pain typically responds to treatment (3–10 days) before depressive symptoms (2–4 weeks), and at doses one-third to one-half of those needed to treat depression.

Bupropion SR (sustained-release), a dopamine and norepinephrine reuptake inhibitor, and venlafaxine, a serotonin and norepinephrine reuptake inhibitor, produced significant improvement in neuropathic pain and/or DPNP compared with placebo.[11–13] Selective serotonin reuptake inhibitors (SSRIs) can alleviate pain in depressed patients, but they are less effective in treating pain in non-depressed patients, perhaps due to their selectivity for serotonin.[14] Further, recent FDA warnings suggest that SSRIs may be associated with suicidal ideations, particularly in depressed adolescents, and all patients started on SSRIs should be regularly evaluated for suicidal thinking.

Anticonvulsants

Pregabalin is the only anticonvulsant available in the USA with a labeled indication for the treatment of DPNP.[15] It is an analog of γ-aminobutyric acid (GABA). It binds to calcium channels, and modulates presynaptic release of excitatory neurotransmitters.[16] Several large trials have demonstrated the efficacy of pregabalin to lower pain scores and reduce sleep interference.[17] In these trials, patients also reported less tension and anxiety, and mood symptoms improved as well.

Carbamazepine was one of the first anticonvulsant medications used for DPNP. It is chemically similar to TCAs and is as effective as nortriptyline for relieving pain.[18] Common side effects of carbamazepine are dose-related and can be minimized by starting with a low dose (100 mg/day). Blood dyscrasias (agranulocytosis and aplastic anemia) do occur with increased frequency, are idiosyncratic and the incidence is highest during the first 3 months of treatment. A complete blood count (CBC) is monitored 2–4 weeks after starting therapy and then every 3–6 months thereafter. If the white blood cell (WBC) count drops below 3000/mm^3, or the absolute neutrophil count is 1000/mm^3, the medication should be tapered and stopped. Electrolytes and liver function tests should be obtained at baseline, and monitored because carbamazepine is also associated with the syndrome of inappropriate antidiuretic hormone (SIADH) secretion and hepatotoxicity. Oxcarbazepine, related chemically to carbamazepine, has shown efficacy in a 9-week, open-label trial with patients having DPNP.[19] Unlike carbamazepine, oxcarbazepine has no bone marrow suppression or hepatotoxicity, and, in general, has a better side-effect profile.

Gabapentin and lamotrigine significantly decrease pain in patients with DPN.[20–22] Gabapentin also improves sleep, and quality of life, and has similar efficacy to that of TCAs and carbamazepine. Patients usually develop tolerance to dizziness associated with gabapentin. Lamotrigine is started at 50 mg/day for 2 weeks and increased to 50 mg/day for 2 weeks; then weekly increases of 100 mg/day may be made based on treatment response. Serious adverse effects, such as Stevens–Johnson syndrome and angioedema, occur rarely (0.3%). The concomitant use of valproic acid and lamotrigine, initiating lamotrigine at too high a dose, and rapidly increasing the dose, are associated with these serious adverse effects.

In a small sample of patients, 60% of whom had DPNP, the combination of morphine and gabapentin produced greater pain relief at lower doses of each drug than either medication used as a single agent. Constipation, sedation, and dry mouth occurred with greater frequency with combined treatment than with either agent alone.[23]

Maximum tolerated doses for morphine and gabapentin in combination were lower than for each medication when used alone.

Topiramate has been shown to reduce pain scores by 30% in half of treated patients with diabetes in one study but not in others.[24] A syndrome consisting of acute myopia associated with secondary angle closure glaucoma has been reported in patients receiving topiramate. Symptoms include acute onset of decreased visual acuity and/or ocular pain occurring within 1 month of initiating therapy. In contrast to primary narrow angle glaucoma, which is rare under 40 years of age, secondary angle closure glaucoma associated with topiramate has been reported in children as well as adults. Topiramate should be discontinued immediately, and the patient referred to an ophthalmologist. There is insufficient evidence to support the use of phenytoin, valproic acid, or levetiracetam for DPNP.

Opioids

Pain should be managed whenever it occurs. There is no justification for holding off therapy until pain is worse when many treatments are available for the control of DPNP. Nowhere is there more concern expressed about this issue than in connection with the prescription of opiates. This, in conjunction with worries about the abuse potential of this class of medication have led to the development of 'universal precautions' in pain management when opioids are prescribed for extended periods of time[25,26] (Table 11.2).

Several double-blind, randomized controlled trials (RCTs) have shown efficacy for oxycodone controlled-release (CR), morphine, and methadone in diabetic and post-herpetic neuropathic pain.[27–29] Oxycodone CR formulations have been effective for DPNP[27,28] and better tolerated than TCAs for neuropathic pain in those patients who continued taking medication.[27] Additionally, oxycodone CR gave greater pain intensity improvement, with lower mean daily pain, steady pain, and brief pain scores compared with active placebo ($p = 0.0001$ for all).[28] The usual starting dose of oxycodone CR is 10 mg every 12 hours (equivalent to taking four 5 mg doses of oxycodone daily), which is then increased up to as much as 40–60 mg/day in two doses given 12 hours apart. Oxycodone CR may be asymmetrically dosed, given as two different doses 12 hours apart, if pain is more bothersome during some parts of the day than others (night vs day).

Table 11.2 The key aspects of long-term opioid management

- A thorough history and physical examination
- Determination of the etiology of the pain
- Establishment of the diagnosis
- Identification of risk factors for substance abuse before starting long-term opioid therapy
- Documentation of observations and clinical findings objectively
- Informed consent from the patient before opioid therapy is started, so there is no doubt about the treatment proposed or the outcome expected
- A written opioid treatment agreement that defines the expectations and obligations for the patient and the provider
- Patient agreement to use only one provider and one pharmacy for opioids
- Ongoing administration of pre- and post-intervention assessments of pain intensity and function
- Monitoring of the emergence of adverse effects or aberrant behavior
- Prescriptions of long-acting opioid analgesics are on a time-contingent basis
- Use of 'rational polypharmacy' that includes adjuvants with opioids
- Use of the minimum effective dose necessary to maintain function
- Periodic urine drug screens to rule out medication diversion and identify use of illicit substances
- Periodic assessment for development of addiction

Using this dosing strategy can significantly reduce the risk of respiratory depression, which many clinicians needlessly fear. The common side effects initially experienced include nausea, constipation, increased sweating, and sedation. Whereas many clinicians may fear respiratory depression, using the above-mentioned dosing strategy, over time, tolerance develops to the early side effects except for constipation. With ongoing treatment, lowering of sexual hormone levels may become a long-term issue, leading to erectile dysfunction for men and amenorrhea for women.

Methadone is a potent μ opioid receptor agonist. The properties of this drug set it apart from other opioids, such that it is recommended as the first-line opioid of choice for DPNP. It currently has no regulatory approval or license for this indication. These properties include:

- *N*-methy 1-*D* aspartate (NMDA)-receptor antagonism
- norepinephrine and serotonin reuptake inhibition
- trimodal metabolism and excretion (hepatic, fecal, and renal)
- no clinically significant metabolites
- high bioavailability
- low cost.[30]

Methadone administration requires patience and frequent initial dose adjustments. Patients who are candidates for methadone treatment are those who have failed to respond to medication trials of maximized doses of non-narcotics (antidepressants, anticonvulsants) and who are experiencing moderate to severe pain. Patients are generally started on 2.5–5 mg every 8 hours. Since diabetic pain is often worse at night, a larger dose may be needed at bedtime, or during times of the day when the pain is more intense. Upward titration occurs every 4–7 days, depending on analgesic response and need for breakthrough pain dosing. Some patients may need 6-hour dosing schedules. Breakthrough doses should be 10–20% of the total daily dose, given every 3–4 hours. Frail elderly patients should be started on 0.5–1 mg every 8 hours, with slower dose titration.

Conversion to methadone from other opioids is non-linear, so that the larger the dose of opioid, the smaller the conversion ratio will be to methadone (3:1 for <100 mg/day of morphine-equivalents, but 20:1 for >1000 mg/day morphine-equivalents).[31] When converting, clinicians should use a methadone conversion table after first obtaining the morphine-equivalent dose.[30] The initial starting dose of methadone should be decreased by 25–50% because cross-tolerance is often incomplete.

Side effects, which include nausea, vomiting, pruritus, and sweating, are generally managed with dose reductions of ~25%. Constipation, the most common side effect, will need aggressive intervention, and may require stool softeners as well as dietary considerations (fresh vegetables, fruit, water, fiber) and exercise.

Tramadol, a centrally acting μ opioid agonist, is also a weak inhibitor of norepinephrine and serotonin reuptake. It has been shown in a placebo-controlled RCT to be significantly more effective than placebo for DPNP ($p < 0.001$), improving paresthesias ($p = 0.001$), and touch-evoked pain ($p = 0.001$). NNT with tramadol were 3.1–4.3.[32–34] Treatment is started at 50 mg/day, and increased by 50 mg every 3–5 days. Effective doses range between 100 and 400 mg/day, usually in divided doses. Common side effects include dizziness, vertigo, nausea, constipation, headache, and somnolence. Patients at risk for seizures should avoid use of this drug. There is also a risk for serotonin syndrome in patients who are concomitantly treated with SSRIs.

Topical agents

Topical agents work locally at the site of application with little systemic effect. The mechanism of action of lidocaine is inhibition of voltage-gated sodium channels. The 5% lidocaine patch has demonstrated efficacy in DPNP, with the NNT comparable to other available treatments.[35,36] The patch may be worn up to 12 hours daily, with up to three patches used together.[37]

Capsaicin, the alkaloid found in hot peppers, depletes tissue substance P and reduces chemically triggered pain. Capsaicin cream must be applied four times daily, often to large surface areas, initially producing unpleasant burning sensations that may be intolerable for some patients; it requires weeks of consistent use to be most effective.[38] Capsaicin cream is best used for those with localized rather than widespread neuropathic pain.[38]

Non-pharmacologic interventions

Although certainly not conventional therapy, when treatment for DPNP is ineffective or linked to unacceptable side effects, spinal cord stimulation (SCS) may be another option. There have been no large studies using SCS (with the insertion of electrical leads, wires, and generator/battery packs into the bodies of people with hyperglycemia posing potential serious risk of nervous system infection). In one small study with 10 patients who had intractable DPNP, SCS gave eight of them statistically significant background and peak pain level reductions, with improvement in their exercise tolerance.[39] There are currently no data to support the use of an implanted medication delivery system (pump) and a tunneled catheter into the epidural or subarachnoid spaces in DPNP.

Stimulation-produced analgesia (SPA), whether performed by electrical means or manually, provides analgesia through the release of endogenous opioid-like molecules and gives temporary relief of pain, but long-term pain reduction is not clearly established.[34] Transcutaneous electrical nerve stimulation (TENS) reportedly gives pain relief during treatment, but has very low residual effects.[34] TENS can enhance endogenous opioids with the A-mode (low frequency with wide pulse width) if the patient is not using exogenous opioid medications. Using the C-mode (high frequency with narrow pulse width) gives local comfort similar to licking or rubbing a painful area after injury. Percutaneous electrical nerve stimulation (PENS) is the delivery of electrical energy through acupuncture needles inserted through the skin. PENS can lessen impedance from the skin, reportedly producing pain relief, increasing activity, and improving sleep.[34] Acupuncture, the placement of needles into specific points along 'energy pathways' (meridians) to 'sedate' or 'tonify' them, reportedly produces benefits lasting more than 6 months and reduces the use of other analgesics.[40] Most of these types of treatments are provided by physical therapists (TENS), acupuncturists, and chiropractors (acupuncture and PENS). Controlled trials are lsimited, comparison of results is difficult, and operator issues (standard acupuncture regimen [SAR] vs traditional Chinese medicine [TCM]) add to the confusion about these techniques for DPNP.

Frequency-modulated electromagnetic neural stimulation (FREMS) lowered pain scores ($p < 0.02$) for patients receiving two series (10 treatments) lasting no more than 3 weeks. FREMS also increased sensory tactile perception as assessed by monofilament testing, and increased motor conduction velocity when compared with placebo (all $p < 0.01$).[41]

More controversial than other 'alternative' therapies, the wearing of magnetic insoles has been reported to lessen DPNP. Subjects ($n = 375$) with stage II or III DPN were assigned to wear magnetized insoles for 4 months. There were statistically significant reductions during the third and fourth months in burning, numbness, tingling, and exercise-induced foot pain ($p < 0.05$ for all). The authors concluded that static magnetic fields penetrate up to 20 mm in depth and target ectopic firing nociceptors with analgesic benefits achieved over time.[42]

Disease-modifying treatments

Presently, disease-modifying approaches have yet to be proven beneficial, but remain an area of focus for investigation.[34] Treatment with angiotensin-converting enzyme (ACE) inhibitors improves electrophysiologic nerve function, but its clinical relevance is unknown. A meta-analysis of RCTs of aldose reductase (AR) inhibitors has demonstrated beneficial effects on motor, but not sensory, nerves. The degree of AR inhibition may be an important factor in improvement of sensory nerves, however. A recent study found dose-dependent improvements in symptoms of numbness, pain, paresthesias, and hyperesthesia, in 279 diabetic patients.[43] To date, only one country (Japan) has approved an AR inhibitor for this indication.

With oxidative stress playing a role in DPN, trials of the antioxidant α-lipoic acid (ALA), a powerful oxygen radical scavenger which regenerates glutathione,[43] have been conducted. Doses of ALA ranged from 600 to 1200 mg/day, but results have been varied.[44,45] Evening primrose oil is a highly concentrated omega-6 fatty acid rich in γ-linolenic acid (GLA), essential for nerve health and myelin integrity.[46] GLA-treated patients with DPNP had significant improvement in nerve function tests in one study, and no improvement in vibratory threshold in another study.[47,48]

Best practices

In 2005, a group of pain management experts developed treatment recommendations for DPN, which resulted in the ranking of currently available therapies. The criteria used to make these categorizations included:

- two or more RCTs in DPN to be deemed a first-line therapy
- one or more RCT in DPN or another neuropathic pain state to be deemed a second-line therapy
- some mechanism of action suggesting potential efficacy for DPN
- one or more RCT for another pain state for 'honorable mention' status.

The consensus of the advisory group was that duloxetine, oxycodone CR, pregabalin, and the entire class of TCAs were all first-line agents for the treatment of DPN. Second-line therapies for DPN included carbamazepine, gabapentin, lamotrigine, tramadol, and venlafaxine ER (extended-release). Honorable mentions went to bupropion, capsaicin, citalopram, lidocaine, methadone, paroxetine, phenytoin, and topiramate. The role of acupuncture, electrical stimulation, magnetic therapy, implanted medication delivery systems, meditation and prayer, SCS, and several other therapies was not considered by the group.

Summary

DPN is a condition that affects many persons with DM, and at times causes significant pain and disability, as well as being a leading cause of foot ulcers that contribute to non-traumatic amputations. Risk factors for DPN include duration of diabetes, poor glycemic control, vascular disease, age, obesity, and height. Treatment consists of prevention and symptom management. Providers must screen for early manifestations of DM and of DPN to detect sensory changes and prevent foot injury. The clinician and patient must establish a common understanding of realistic, quantifiable pain treatment goals. Time-limited trials of medications, alone or in combination, are warranted for pain relief, and most patients will experience significant pain relief most of the time.

References

1. National Diabetes Education Program (NDEP). Take care of your feet for a lifetime. Available at: http://www.ndep.nih.gov/diabetes/pubs/FootTips.pdf. Accessed on 1/23/2006.
2. Goldstein DJ, Lu Y, Detke MJ et al. Duloxetine vs. placebo in patients with painful diabetic neuropathy. Pain 2005; 116: 1–10.
3. Raskin J, Pritchett YL, Wang F et al. A double-blind, randomized multicenter trial comparing duloxetine with placebo in the management of diabetic peripheral neuropathic pain. Pain Med 2005; 6: 346–56.
4. Chen H, Lamer TJ, Rho RH et al. Contemporary management of neuropathic pain for the primary care physician. Mayo Clin Proc 2004; 79: 1533–45.
5. Barbano R, Hart-Gouleau S, Pennella-Vaughan J, Dworkin RH. Pharmacotherapy of painful diabetic neuropathy. Curr Pain Headache Rep 2003; 7: 169–77.
6. Dworkin RH, Backonja M, Rowbotham MC et al. Advances in neuropathic pain: diagnosis, mechanisms, and treatment recommendations. Arch Neurol 2003; 60(11): 1524–34.
7. Max MB, Culnane M, Schafer SC et al. Amitriptyline relieves diabetic neuropathic pain in patients with normal or depressed mood. Neurology 1987; 37: 589–96.
8. Kvinesdal B, Molin J, Froland A, Gram LF. Imipramine treatment of painful diabetic neuropathy. JAMA 1984; 251: 1727–30.
9. Max MB, Kishore-Kumar R, Schafer SC et al. Efficacy of desipramine in painful diabetic neuropathy: a placebo controlled trial. Pain 1991; 45: 3–9.
10. Max MB, Lynch SA, Muir J et al. Effects of desipramine, amitriptyline and fluoxetine on pain in diabetic neuropathy. N Engl J Med 1992; 326: 1250–6.
11. Semenchuk MR, Sherman R, Davis B. Double-blind, randomized trial of bupropion SR for the treatment of neuropathic pain. Neurology 2001; 57: 1583–8.
12. Sindrup SH, Bach FW, Madsen C et al. Venlafaxine versus imipramine in painful polyneuropathy: a randomized, controlled trial. Neurology 2003; 60: 1284–9.
13. Rowbotham MC, Goli V, Kunz NR, Lei D. Venlafaxine extended release in the treatment of painful diabetic neuropathy: a double-blind, placebo-controlled study. Pain 2004; 110: 697–706.
14. Goodnick PJ. Use of antidepressants in treatment of comorbid diabetes mellitus and depression as well as in diabetic neuropathy. Ann Clin Psychiatry 2001; 13(1): 31–41.

15. Backonja M-M. Pregabalin in painful diabetic peripheral neuropathy. Drugs 2004; 64: 2821.

16. Frampton JE, Foster RH. Pregabalin: in the treatment of postherpetic neuralgia. Drugs 2005; 65: 111–18.

17. Rosenstock J, Tuchman M, LaMoreaux L, Sharma U. Pregabalin for the treatment of painful diabetic peripheral neuropathy: a double-blind, placebo-controlled trial. Pain 2004; 110: 628–38.

18. Gomez-Perez FJ, Choza R, Rios JM et al. Nortriptyline-fluphenazine vs. carbamazepine in the symptomatic treatment of diabetic neuropathy. Arch Med Res 1996; 27: 525–9.

19. Beydoun A, Kobetz SA, Carrazana EJ. Efficacy of oxcarbazepine in the treatment of painful diabetic neuropathy. Clin J Pain 2004; 20: 174–8.

20. Backonja M-M, Beydoun A, Edwards KR et al. Gabapentin for the treatment of painful neuropathy in patients with diabetes mellitus: a randomized controlled trial. JAMA 1998; 280: 1831–6.

21. Gorson KC, Schott C, Herman R, Ropper AH, Rand WM. Gabapentin in the treatment of painful diabetic neuropathy: a placebo controlled, double blind, crossover trial. J Neurol Neurosurg Psychiatry 1999; 66: 251–2.

22. Eisenberg E, Lurie Y, Braker C, Daoud D, Ishay A. Lamotrigine reduces painful diabetic neuropathy: a randomized, controlled study. Neurology 2001; 57: 505–9.

23. Gilron I, Bailey JM, Tu D et al. Morphine, gabapentin, or their combination for neuropathic pain. N Engl J Med 2005; 352: 1324–34.

24. Raskin P, Donofrio PD, Rosenthal NR et al, for the CAPSS-141 Study Group. Topiramate vs placebo in painful diabetic neuropathy: analgesic and metabolic effects. Neurology 2004; 63: 865–73.

25. Gourlay DL, Heit HA, Almahrezi A. Universal precautions in pain medicine: a rational approach to the treatment of chronic pain. Pain Med 2005; 6(2): 107–12.

26. Cole BE. Prescribing opioids, relieving patient suffering, and staying out of personal trouble with regulators: reprising old ideas and offering new suggestions. Pain Pract 2002; 12: 5–8. Available at: http://www.aapainmanage.org/literature/PainPrac/V12N3_Cole_PrescribingOpioids.pdf. Accessed on 1/23/2006.

27. Gimbel JS, Richards P, Portenoy RK. Controlled-release oxycodone for pain in diabetic neuropathy: a randomized controlled trial. Neurology 2003; 60: 927–43.

28. Watson CPN, Moulin D, Watt-Watson J, Gordon A, Eisenhoffer J. Controlled-release oxycodone relieves neuropathic pain: a randomized controlled trial in painful diabetic neuropathy. Pain 2003; 105: 71–8.

29. Raja SN, Haythornthwaite JA, Pappagallo M et al. Opioids versus antidepressants in postherpetic neuralgia: a randomized, placebo-controlled trial. Neurology 2002; 59: 1015–21.

30. Hays L, Ried C, Doran M, Geary K. Use of methadone for the treatment of diabetic neuropathy. Diabetes Care 2005; 28: 485–7.

31. Gazelle G, Fine PG. Fast fact and concept #075: methadone for pain. End-of-Life Physician Education Resource Center. Available at: http://www.eperc.mcw.edu/fastFact/ff_75.htm. Accessed on 1/23/2006.

32. Harati Y, Gooch C, Swenson M et al. Double-blind randomized trial of tramadol for the treatment of the pain of diabetic neuropathy. Neurology 1998; 50: 1842–6.

33. Sindrup SH, Anderson G, Madsen C et al. Tramadol relieves pain and allodynia in polyneuropathy: a randomized, double-blind, controlled trial. Pain 1999; 83: 85–90.

34. Duby JJ, Campbell RK, Setter SM, White JR, Rasmussen KA. Diabetic neuropathy: an intensive review. Am J Health Syst Pharm 2004; 61: 160–76.

35. Argoff CE, Galer BS, Jensen MP, Oleka N, Gammaitoni AR. Effectiveness of the lidocaine patch 5% on pain qualities in three chronic pain states: assessment with the Neuropathic Pain Scale. Curr Med Res Opin 2004; 20(Suppl 2): S21–S28.

36. Meier T, Wasner G, Faust M et al. Efficacy of lidocaine patch 5% in the treatment of focal peripheral neuropathic pain syndromes: a randomized, double-blind, placebo-controlled study. Pain 2003; 106; 151–8.

37. Pasero C. Lidocaine patch 5%. Am J Nurs 2003; 103: 75–7.

38. Boulton AJM. Management of diabetic peripheral neuropathy. Clin Diabetes 2005; 23: 9–15. Available at:
http://clinical.diabetesjournals.org/cgi/content/abstract/23/1/9.
Accessed on 1/17/2006.

39. Tesfaye S, Watt J, Benbow SJ et al. Electrical spinal-cord stimulation for painful diabetic peripheral neuropathy. Lancet 1996; 348: 1698–1701.

40. Abuaisha BB, Costanzi JB, Boulton AJ. Acupuncture for the treatment of chronic painful diabetic neuropathy: a long-term study. Diabetes Res Clin Pract 1998; 39: 115–21.

41. Bosi E, Conti M, Vermigli C et al. Effectiveness of frequency-modulated electromagnetic neural stimulation in the treatment of painful diabetic neuropathy. Diabetologia 2005; 48: 817–23.

42. Weintraub MI, Wolfe GI, Barohn RA et al. Static magnetic field therapy for symptomatic diabetic neuropathy: a randomized, double-blind, placebo-controlled trial. Arch Phys Med Rehabil 2003; 84: 736–46.

43. Boulton AJM, Malik RA, Arezzo JC, Sosenko JM. Diabetic somatic neuropathies. Diabetes Care 2004; 27: 1458–86.

44. Ziegler D, Hanefeld M, Ruhnau KJ et al. Treatment of symptomatic diabetic peripheral neuropathy with the antioxidant alpha-lipoic acid. A 3-week multicenter, randomized controlled trial (ALADIN Study). Diabetologia 1995; 38: 1425–33.

45. Ziegler D, Hanefeld M, Ruhnau KJ et al. Treatment of symptomatic diabetic polyneuropathy with the antioxidant alpha-lipoic acid: a 7-month multicenter randomized controlled trial (ALADIN III Study). Diabetes Care 1999; 22: 1296–1301.

46. Halat KM, Dennehy CE. Botanicals and dietary supplements in diabetic peripheral neuropathy. J Am Board Fam Pract 2003; 16: 47–57.

47. Keen H, Payan J, Allawi J et al. Treatment of diabetic neuropathy with gamma-linolenic acid. Diabetes Care 1993; 16: 8–15.

48. Purewal TS, Evans PMS, Havard F, O'Hare JP. Lack of effect of evening primrose oil on autonomic function tests after 12 months of treatment. Diabetologia 1997; 40(Suppl 1): A556.

Chapter 12

Psychosocial therapies for psychiatric disorders and diabetes mellitus

Alan M Delamater, Jessica M Valenzuela, and Michelle M Castro

Introduction

A substantial amount of research has established the significant role of psychosocial factors in diabetes management.[1] Many patients have great difficulty with the diagnosis of diabetes, and beyond the psychologic challenges of disease adaptation, many develop psychiatric disorders over the course of diabetes. To the extent they do, such disorders may compromise the ability of patients to effectively manage diabetes. In this chapter, we review the evidence regarding the more common psychiatric disorders affecting individuals with diabetes mellitus (DM), including depression, anxiety disorders, and eating disorders. Our focus is on describing and evaluating psychosocial therapies for psychiatric disorders among patients with DM, including both type 1 and type 2 DM. We first consider the literature regarding adults, and then focus on research studies conducted with children. While many studies have addressed the role of psychosocial factors in diabetes management, fewer have addressed psychosocial therapies for specific psychiatric disorders.

Psychosocial interventions in adults with diabetes mellitus

Depression

There is strong evidence that depression is more prevalent in patients with DM,[2] associated with poor adherence,[2] higher rates of hyperglycemia,[3] and a higher risk of complications in individuals with DM.[4] A recent meta-analysis indicated that adults with DM have an increased prevalence of depression and other psychiatric disorders than their healthy counterparts.[5] Given that depression is a prevalent and significant risk factor for poor health outcomes, it is surprising that few controlled studies of psychosocial interventions in this population exist.

Both cognitive and behavioral therapies are well-established empirically supported treatments for depression in the general population.[6] Cognitive behavioral therapy (CBT) is the treatment of choice for many counselors and therapists, and no other psychosocial intervention has been as thoroughly investigated across a variety of disorders. In addition to being well studied and effective, CBT interventions can be brief, group-based, structured, and manual-driven. Consequently, CBT is often favored by insurance companies and managed care organizations. On the one hand, therapists working with this population should use CBT to address diabetes-related stressors such as feelings and thoughts of guilt, anger, or loss of control surrounding the development of complications.[7] Still, therapy should also be patient-focused and should evaluate the patient's general life stressors, such as work, finances, and relationships, as these contribute significantly to psychological distress in individuals with DM.[8] Several studies have examined the effects of CBT in individuals who have not been diagnosed with any psychiatric disorder, and these generally have shown reductions in diabetes-related stress and improvements in quality of life after treatment.

To date, there has been only one randomized controlled trial (RCT) of CBT in adults with comorbid type 2 DM and diagnosed depression. Lustman and colleagues tested a 10-week group CBT intervention.[9] The group sessions focused on behavior change, problem-solving, and recognizing maladaptive cognitions. Despite a small sample size, the researchers found that CBT alongside diabetes education leads to a 75–85% depression remission rate and offers an advantage over diabetes education alone in treating individuals with type 2 DM and depression. In addition to improving depressive symptoms, they found that CBT was associated with improved glycemic control (9.5% compared with 10.9% in the control group). Depression treatment may improve glycemic control through improved regimen adherence or through physiologic means, such as changes in stress-related hormones that can affect glycemic control.[10] More research is needed to clarify the relationship between depression treatment and glycemic control.

Medical factors associated with DM affected patient response to CBT. Individuals with lower compliance to blood glucose monitoring, higher glycosylated hemoglobin levels, greater weight, and more diabetes-related complications had diminished response to treatment.[11] These findings suggest that for psychotherapy to be effective, therapists need to work as part of a health care team. Collaboration with physicians, nurse practitioners, nutritionists, and other health care professionals is necessary in order for therapists to achieve the best possible treatment response.

Over the past 20 years, interpersonal therapy (IPT) has been established as an empirically supported treatment in depression in the general population.[6] Several large RCTs support the efficacy of IPT in treating depression. It is a short-term manualized therapy that can be used for treatment of depression and for maintenance of treatment effects.[12] IPT addresses relational issues surrounding depression in one of four areas: interpersonal disputes, role transitions, grief, or interpersonal deficit. Although there have been no published studies focusing on IPT in people with DM, Rubin and Peyrot suggest that it may be a useful intervention tool with this population.[13] Individuals with DM may especially benefit from IPT techniques such as communication analysis and training, role-playing interpersonal scenarios, and problem-solving, because of the multiple interactions with health care professionals and others surrounding their illness. Studies looking at IPT in comorbid DM and depression are needed.

There have been two large-scale trials of 'collaborative care' in multiple primary care clinics treating patients with diabetes. In this case, collaborative care includes either antidepressant medication or problem-solving therapy (PST). PST consists of seven stages whereby patients are encouraged to apply problem-solving skills to at least one problem per treatment session.[14] The Pathways Study randomized diabetic participants with depressed mood to either a usual care–control condition or an intervention which allowed patients to choose medication or PST.[15] Patients in the intervention condition whose symptoms persisted after 10–12 weeks were allowed to change medications or mode of treatment. In addition, if symptoms persisted after another 8–12 weeks, patients were referred to specialty care. The IMPACT trial compared usual care and a similar intervention in diabetic adults >60 years old.[16] These trials found that collaborative 'stepped' care in a primary care setting improves depression severity, adequacy of self-administering antidepressant medications, satisfaction with care, and, in older adults, functional status.

Two controlled trials randomized depressed adults with comorbid DM to treatment with antidepressants.[17,18] Both tricyclic antidepressants and selective serotonin reuptake inhibitors (SSRIs) were found to improve depressive symptoms compared with placebo in type 1 and type 2 DM. However, tricyclic antidepressants had a hyperglycemic effect detrimental to glycemic control.[18] Musselman and others have suggested that antidepressant medication alone should be considered before psychosocial interventions or combined therapy, because people with DM have complicated regimens.[10] They consider antidepressant medication to be the least effortful intervention. However, combination therapy with CBT and antidepressant medication is considered an excellent intervention tool to treat depression. It is significantly more effective than either intervention alone in the general population.[19] More research is needed to determine the acceptability and effectiveness of combination therapy in adults with DM and depression.

There is some evidence that the present quality of care for patients with DM and major depression is less than satisfactory. Often, diabetic patients are prescribed very low doses of antidepressant medications and discontinued from treatment even though they are at high risk for relapse.[20] In addition, there is evidence that few patients receive even four psychotherapy visits after being diagnosed with depression.[15] Researchers have suggested that reform is needed in five specific areas:

- identification of individuals with comorbid DM and depression
- monitoring of patients between appointments
- better coordination efforts among health care professionals
- increased access to therapy
- additional emphasis on physical activity.[21]

From the data available it appears that antidepressant medications and CBT have a similar response rate in DM as in the general population. Furthermore, patient-centered collaborative care with 'stepped care' for patients with persistent symptoms is a promising intervention model in primary care settings. More trials are needed, however, to increase confidence in the reliability, generalizability, and feasibility of these findings, as well as to explore other possibly useful interventions in this population, such as IPT.

Stress and anxiety disorders

Cognitive behavioral therapies are among the best-studied interventions for anxiety disorders in the general population. CBT is considered a 'well-established' treatment for panic disorder, agoraphobia, and generalized anxiety disorder. In addition, exposure treatment is a 'well-established' treatment for specific phobia, agoraphobia, and obsessive-compulsive disorder.[6] There are also many interventions that can be considered 'probably efficacious' in treating anxiety disorders (e.g. progressive muscular relaxation, EMDR [eye movement densensitization and reprocessing] for post-traumatic stress disorder, etc.). There have been few studies, however, addressing the treatment of anxiety disorders in patients with diabetes.

Due to the possible deleterious effects of stress and anxiety on metabolic activity, reviewed in Surwit and Schneider,[22] researchers have studied the effects of biofeedback-assisted relaxation training (BFRT) and progressive relaxation training interventions on glycemic control in individuals with type 2 DM.[23–28] Alternative kinds of relaxation interventions have also been effective in improving glycemic control. For example, a recent study showed improved insulin resistance after a traditional Chinese relaxation exercise named Qigong.[29] While these studies focus primarily on the effects of relaxation on insulin resistance and do not include assessment of clinically significant anxiety symptoms, several studies show moderate improvements in state and trait anxiety scores for patients trained in relaxation interventions.[24,26,27,29]

There is a debate as to whether baseline anxiety levels predict response to stress management interventions. Some studies indicate that distressed and anxious patients benefit the least from the possible improvements in glycemic control that are sometimes associated with these interventions.[23,27] Yet a recent study by Surwit et al indicated no difference in treatment response.[28] As long as data in this area are controversial, it may be helpful for patients with significant anxiety to be treated with medication or CBT prior to relaxation interventions, in order to optimize the results of these interventions on blood glucose.[27]

Anxiety medications such as benzodiazepines and SSRIs can be effective in the treatment of anxiety disorders, but have not been well studied in adults with DM.[13] Likewise, there is limited research on psychotherapy in individuals diagnosed with DM and a comorbid anxiety disorder. Data looking at anxiety symptoms and diabetes-related stress in non-clinical samples have provided accumulating evidence that CBT can effectively aid in reducing these symptoms. A recent study in Norway demonstrated reduced DM-related stress and improved coping in individuals with both types of DM after an intensive group-based CBT program.[30] These groups were led by specialist nurses and experienced individuals with DM who had been trained in a 16-hour course. Individuals with type 1 and type 2 DM constituted different subgroups. There were nine group sessions which focused largely on problem-solving and decision-making, as well as cognitive restructuring. Intervention effects were maintained at the 12-month follow-up. Older studies including people with both type 1 and type 2 DM also show reduced anxiety levels after cognitive behavioral stress-reduction interventions.[31-33]

Anxious individuals with diabetes may be susceptible to significant fears of hypoglycemia, injections, and/or diabetes-related complications. The literature indicates that these fears are associated with poor adherence[34,35] and may lead to an increased risk of complications.[36] In fact, there is evidence that anxiety symptoms are specifically related to injection avoidance in people with diabetes.[37] These issues highlight the importance of interventions to reduce anxiety symptoms in this population. Case studies that include clinically anxious individuals with diabetes indicate that CBT can be effective in reducing panic attacks, avoidance behaviors, and fear of hypoglycemia.[38,39] These interventions included the following components:

- elimination of safety behaviors, such as eating to prevent hypoglycemia before checking for low blood sugar
- creation of a fear hierarchy
- exposure to feared stimuli, including exposure to an induced hypoglycemic episode
- instruction on relaxation/distraction techniques.

It is also important to note that it may be important for mental health professionals working with this comorbid population to have specific knowledge in the area of DM and to work closely as a part of the patient's medical team. For example, difficulty discriminating between anxiety symptoms and an actual hypoglycemic episode can be difficult for both patients and therapists.[40,41] In such a situation, it could be dangerous for a therapist to train the individual in CBT or relaxation techniques, because of the danger inherent in minimizing an actual hypoglycemic episode. Thus, close collaboration with the health care team is essential.

Eating disorders in adolescent girls and women

Prevalence rates of eating disorders, including anorexia, bulimia, binge-eating disorder (BED), and eating disorders not otherwise specified (ED-NOS), have been shown to be 5.4–7% in women with type 1 DM (lifetime 10.5–14.4%) and 6.5–9% in women with type 2 DM (lifetime 10–13.7%).[42] In fact, eating disorders are twice as common in adolescent females with type 1 DM as in non-diabetic adolescents.[43] Some researchers suggest that this increased prevalence of eating disorders in the diabetic population may be due to various risk factors associated with the illness. For example, susceptible individuals could develop disordered eating behaviors and attitudes due to rapid weight gain associated with the start of insulin treatment or the increased focus on food and dietary restrictions needed for diabetes self-care. In addition, hunger associated with hypoglycemic episodes may lead to binge-eating behaviors.[44]

Whereas Herpertz et al[42] found no difference in the prevalence of eating disorders between people with type 1 and type 2 DM, they did find a difference in the distribution of specific eating disorders. In individuals with type 1 DM, the prevalence of different eating disorders was fairly consistent. Also, individuals with type 1 DM were more likely to develop an eating disorder after the onset of diabetes. In contrast, individuals with type 2 DM were disproportionately more likely to be diagnosed with BED than any other eating disorder, and more frequently had an eating disorder that preceded their diagnosis with DM, suggesting that individuals may develop type 2 DM as a consequence of an eating disorder.

In the general population, CBT is considered a probably efficacious treatment for BED and bulimia. IPT has also been shown to be valuable in the treatment of bulimia nervosa.[6,45] In anorexia nervosa, researchers have shown successful application of CBT and have suggested that a family therapy component is also indicated.[46] However, the diagnosis and treatment of disturbed eating attitudes in people with DM can be complex. Health care professionals must have an understanding of the normal focus of food and eating that is a part of DM management in order to determine if their patients have abnormal eating concerns or behaviors.[13]

In type 1 DM, these comorbid conditions may lead to unique purging behaviors such as insulin reduction or omission and unique health care problems such as serious hypoglycemia if eating is restricted. Several studies have focused on insulin omission. Along with a tendency towards disturbed eating attitudes and reporting previous symptoms of anorexia and bulimia, young women who omit insulin also tend to report negative attitudes about diabetes and increased lying to their physician's about their self-management.[47] In addition, insulin-omitters have poorer glycemic control, poorer regimen adherence, and higher rates of retinopathy and neuropathy than non-omitters.[48] As a result, treating disturbed eating attitudes and behaviors in this population is particularly important. However, there are few published treatment studies available.

There are many different levels of treatment possible for comorbid DM and eating disorders: outpatient treatment, intensive outpatient treatment, partial hospitalization, and inpatient hospitalization.[49] Researchers suggest that assessment of severity, type of eating disorder, and managed care considerations should help therapists determine what kinds of treatment to provide.[49,50] For example, more-severe cases may be treated using individual therapy with a psychiatric component, whereas group therapy may be considered in less-severe cases. In addition, Kelly et al[49] suggest a team approach to treatment that includes a physician, dietitian, and a mental health professional. As part of treatment, they propose that the health care team prescribes a less-intensive insulin regimen and less-rigorous nutrition recommendations. These changes are proposed in an effort to decrease the patient's focus on the effects of food, insulin, and exercise on blood glucose. However, the effects of providing a less-intensive regimen in this population have not been studied, and there is the possibility that this could lead to further decline in the glycemic control of these patients. More data are needed on the effects of intensive regimens and treating disturbed-eating attitudes and behaviors.

Older single case-report studies indicate that CBT and integrated approaches, including behavior modification and family interventions, may be effective in females with type 1 DM and anorexia nervosa.[51,52] Also, Rubin and Peyrot suggest that because some antidepressants, such as fluoxetine, paroxetine, and sertraline, have been used to treat compulsive eating behavior in the general population,[13] these medications may be considered for people with DM. However, there are currently no studies on the effects of antidepressants in this particular patient population.

More recently, the role of psychoeducation (PE) with mostly didactic elements has been studied. A randomized study by Olmsted and colleagues, comprising 12–19-year-old girls, showed significant improvements on restraint and eating concerns after a psychoeducational intervention.[53] However, Alloway and colleagues found no improvement with PE in a smaller sample of women with type 1 DM and subclinically disordered eating.[54] A review of group therapies indicates that while educational approaches may change attitudes, they are not successful in changing disturbed eating behaviors.[55]

Takii and colleagues have demonstrated that an integrated inpatient therapy program for treatment of young women with type 1 DM and bulimia can be effective. The inpatient intervention included three components. The first component involved a period of recovery from fatigue and depression. The second component was CBT. Participants worked with a therapist on changing their eating behaviors, diabetes management, and disturbed eating cognitions. The third component of treatment used family counseling to improve family relationships. The intervention led to improvements in eating disorder psychopathology, depressive symptoms, anxiety-proneness, and glycemic control.[56] In type 2 DM, Kenardy and colleagues have shown that cognitive behavioral group therapy improves binge-eating behaviors and disturbed-eating beliefs, and that these benefits can be maintained after intervention.[57] More research is needed in order to learn more about prevention, early intervention, and treatment of eating disorders in both type 1 and 2 DM.

Children and adolescents with diabetes

Prevalence of psychiatric disorders in children and adolescents

Depression

Research suggests that, similar to adults with DM, elevated rates of depression have been found in younger populations. A recent review of the child and adolescent literature revealed an association between

DM and psychological problems, with depression and anxiety the most common psychological disorders.[58] However, the relationship of psychological disorders to glycemic control is not well established.

In three different controlled studies, psychiatric disorders were more prevalent in the diabetes group than in a reference group. When assessing just for depression, there were varied results. Kovacs and colleagues examined the course of depression and found overall rates of recovery and recurrence no different from that of the psychiatric control group.[59] Scores on the Child Depression Inventory (CDI) among the diabetic group were relatively stable, with higher scores appearing at the time of diagnosis of DM and 2 years later. However, at 1-year post diagnosis, no differences were found among groups.[60] Another empirical study concluded that youths with type 1 DM were three times more likely to have a psychiatric disorder.[61] In this study, anxiety and depressive disorders were the most prevalent disorders.

In a 10-year longitudinal study, 26.1% of individuals who developed a psychiatric disorder had suffered from major depression or dysthymia.[62] Additionally, 27.5% were estimated to experience at least one episode of depression by the 10th year. More recently, up to 17% of adolescents reportedly had depressive symptoms, although the true prevalence may vary since the sample was already involved in an intensive management study.[63]

Given the nature of depression, it is not surprising that some studies have assessed the risk of suicide in diabetic patients. In a sample of 95 youths with type 1 DM, 29.5% reported a history of suicidal ideation and 21% had thought about suicide within the last year.[64] Although newly diagnosed patients had elevated rates of ideation, few attempted suicide. The method of attempt was often found to be diabetes-related.

Although several studies have found elevated rates of depression in diabetic youths, two studies reported no differences in psychological well-being among diabetics and youths with other chronic illnesses.[65,66]

Anxiety

Whereas several studies with diabetic youths have examined anxious feelings, there is a scarcity of research on diabetic youths meeting diagnosis of an anxiety disorder. In one longitudinal study, 19.6% of the participants had developed an anxiety disorder by the 10th year, with generalized anxiety disorder being the most common.[62]

Substance abuse

Excessive alcohol consumption and illegal drug use have also been examined in studies of adolescents with DM. Most of the research has focused on the frequency of substance use rather than the incidence of diagnosed substance abuse. Kovacs and colleagues reported in their longitudinal study that 9% of the sample had developed substance abuse disorders by the 10th year after diagnosis of DM.[63] In another study, alcohol consumption was assessed with adolescents at a diabetes summer camp using the Michigan Alcohol Screening Test.[67] Results showed that 24% had abnormal scores. Additionally, 33% of campers reported use of alcohol, 4% marijuana, and 1% cocaine. Glasgow and colleagues found a higher percentage (50%) of adolescents who reported they tried alcohol and about half of those admitted to ongoing use, according to anonymous self-administered questionnaires: one-quarter of them had tried illicit drugs, but only 5% reported still using them.[68] These findings are consistent with other studies that indicate similar rates of alcohol and drug use in diabetic teens.[69]

Psychosocial factors

It is well established that psychosocial factors play an integral role in the management of diabetes in children and adolescents.[1] A number of studies have examined psychological adjustment, self-esteem, and family relationships in children with diabetes. In a study of 91 newly diagnosed children, 33 (36.3%) had developed an adjustment disorder within the first 3 months of diagnosis,[70] but, fortunately, most children's adjustment problems had resolved within the first year after diagnosis. However, in another longitudinal study, psychological adjustment of diabetics was no different 10 years after diagnosis when compared with a group who had moderate to severe acute illnesses.[71] Grey and colleagues found that mild adjustment problems had dissipated by the end of the first year after diagnosis, but some problems reappeared by the end of the second year.[72] Overall, studies indicate that while the majority of children's adjustment problems appear to resolve within the first year, children whose problems do not resolve may be at risk for poor adaptation to DM, including regimen adherence problems, poor metabolic control, and continued psychosocial difficulties.[70-72] Children and adolescents with lower family adaptability, lower family cohesion, and less caring in DM family behaviors were shown to be at greater risk for depressive symptoms than those youths with more adaptive family functioning.[73]

Children with DM may often exhibit symptoms of anxiety related to their diabetes, including fears of injection, hypoglycemia, and health complications.[74-76] Stressors and self-care challenges have also been identified as a common experience of adolescents with type 1 DM.[77]

Adherence, control, and complications

Psychiatric disorders and psychosocial issues

The presence of any psychiatric disorder or psychosocial issue has its own consequences, but for patients with diabetes it often presents an additional barrier to achieving good metabolic control. A recent study by Northam and colleagues showed that 50% of youths with a history of chronic poor glycemic control had a psychiatric diagnosis, whereas only 25% of the well-controlled group had a psychiatric disorder.[78] In another study, adolescents who reported elevated depressive symptoms were twice as likely to be hospitalized due to diabetes-related complications.[79] Other studies indicate that individuals with any psychiatric disorder, including major depression, are at an increased risk for poor glycemic control and development of retinopathy.[70,80] In a recent study reviewing hospital discharge records and diagnoses, adolescents with internalizing disorders had significantly greater risk for repeated hospital admissions, a finding not observed for younger children.[81]

Bryden and colleagues found that scores on the Global Severity Index of mental health predicted recurrent hospitalizations for diabetic ketoacidosis.[82] In a Swedish study, psychological adaptation was the best predictor of metabolic control.[83] Patients with more depressive symptoms experienced poor adaptation, low self-esteem, and poor metabolic control. In contrast, Daviss et al found that depression (measured by the Child Behavior Checklist) did not predict glycemic control; however, glycemic control was predicted by total competence, dietary adherence, and frequency of blood glucose monitoring.[73] Externalizing behavioral problems has also been shown to predict poor glycemic control. In a study by Leonard et al youths with behavioral problems were twice as likely to have HbA$_{1c}$ levels >9% than those without significant behavioral problems.[84]

A number of studies have shown that the family environment and family relationships affect regimen adherence and glycemic control of children and adolescents.[85–88] In a study of the role of parenting styles in young children with DM, parental warmth was predictive of better adherence.[89] Stressful life events, including losses, disappointments, and dangerous experiences were also found to contribute to poor glycemic control.[90] Finally, specific maladaptive coping strategies such as wishful thinking and avoidance have been linked to poor metabolic control.[91–93]

Psychosocial interventions for children and adolescents with diabetes mellitus

Behavioral interventions for youths with type 1 DM tend to be focused on improving self-management and glycemic control, rather than targeted for specific psychiatric disorders. The most common outcome assessed in these interventions, according to a recent meta-analysis, is glycemic control, as measured by HbA_{1c}.[94] Interventions seeking to improve psychosocial outcomes tend to focus on self-efficacy in diabetes management, family conflict (often surrounding the disease), diabetes-specific stress, and/or quality of life measures. These psychosocial interventions have indicated mostly small- to medium-effect sizes.[94]

With the exception of the previously cited literature that targets disturbed eating attitudes in adolescents and young women, few studies focus specifically on intervening with clinically distressed youths. In addition, there is some evidence that exposure to feared stimuli and relaxation/distraction techniques may be effective in reducing significant child distress associated with fear of hypoglycemia or self-injection.[95,96] More research on interventions targeting youths with diabetes who have specific types of psychiatric disorders is clearly needed.

Stress, coping, and problem-solving interventions

Since maladaptive coping strategies and stress seem to contribute to poor diabetic control, it is important to review interventions that may help adolescents develop better coping mechanisms. Theoretically based interventions have been demonstrated to be the most effective.[94] Several intervention studies have incorporated CBT. For example, stress management and coping skills training delivered with small groups of youths has reduced diabetes-related stress[97–99] and improved social interaction.[100] Grey and colleagues[101,102] evaluated the effect of group coping skills training, and found that it improved glycemic control and quality of life for adolescents involved in intensive insulin regimens; effects which were maintained after the intervention was completed.[103] In a peer group intervention study targeting problem-solving, Cook et al found that problem-solving and glucose monitoring increased, whereas glycemic control improved for treated youths.[104] Results of these reports show some promise for the efficacy of group programs utilizing cognitive behavioral stress management interventions for diabetic youths.

Family, peer, and multisystemic interventions

As discussed earlier, there is substantial evidence that family variables, including family conflict, cohesion, and adaptability, are important predictors of regimen adherence and glycemic control in youths with DM. In fact, at least one study has provided evidence that levels of family stress and resources are more strongly related to control than disease-specific variables such as C-peptide levels.[105] Therefore, interventions at the family level have been examined as part of an effort to improve diabetes outcomes. Psychoeducational interventions with children and their families that promote problem-solving skills and increase parental support early in the disease course have been shown to improve long-term glycemic control of children.[106] In a more recent randomized trial, youths who received psychoeducational interventions delivered by a case manager at regular outpatient visits were shown to increase visit frequency, and have reduced acute adverse outcomes such as hypoglycemia and emergency department visits.[107] Because psychosocial and disease-related difficulties in children and adolescents are embedded within other systems, family-centered approaches have been expanded upon to include interventions that target peers and multiple systems, such as a child's community or school.

The 'teamwork' intervention focuses specifically on improving parent–child diabetes-related communication and interactions by encouraging diabetes care responsibility sharing and educating families on ways to avoid parent–child conflict.[108,109] The 'teamwork' intervention is cost-effective, because it can be implemented by paraprofessionals in the family's outpatient diabetes clinic. It has been studied in children 8–16 years old with type 1 DM, and involves three parts: active family discussion and encouragement; written materials; and ongoing negotiation of a family plan. The family discussion and written materials focus on the effects of growth and puberty, the importance of appropriate and supportive parental involvement, coping with and avoiding common family conflict, and realistic expectations for diabetes care, especially daily blood glucose goals. The 'responsibility-sharing' plan highlights specifics about who is responsible for different tasks: e.g. details such as whether or not there will be parental supervision for blood glucose monitoring and how it will be carried out. Like a behavioral contract, this 'responsibility-sharing' plan was encouraged, renegotiated at each session, and reinforced by the family and research assistants. Results from two studies designed to evaluate this office-based intervention show maintenance or improvement of glycemic control.[108,109] In addition, despite increased family involvement, there was stable or reduced family conflict in families who received the intervention compared with a control group.

Multifamily group interventions for diabetes have been shown to have beneficial effects on adherence, control, and perceptions about the disease,[110,111] as well as being perceived by families as acceptable, applicable, and effective in improving general and diabetes-specific family interactions.[112] Wysocki and colleagues have extensively studied the effects of a specific kind of multifamily group intervention,[112–114] behavioral family systems therapy (BFST), on families of adolescents with type 1 DM.[115] BFST includes four components: problem-solving training; communication skills training; cognitive restructuring; and functional/structural family therapy. The revised BFST for DM (BFST-D) also includes (1) targeting two or more diabetes-related problems, (2) inclusion of other social networks such as peers, siblings, and teachers, (3) education about modifying insulin, diet, and exercise based on blood glucose results, (4) detailed behavioral contracting, and (5) parent simulation of living with diabetes, which had been used previous by Satin and colleagues in a multifamily group intervention.[111] Compared with both an educational support group and standard care, BFST-D was associated with less diabetes-related family conflict, improved diabetes self-management, and significantly improved HbA$_{1c}$.[114] Further research is needed to improve the cost-effectiveness and feasibility of BFST-D in this population.

There is considerable evidence that adolescents have more difficulty in managing their DM than younger children, and that declines in glycemic control and adherence are prevalent in early adolescence.[116,117]

In an attempt to create developmentally appropriate interventions for this age group, researchers have developed peer interventions for teens. Greco and colleagues have shown that a peer group intervention, including the best friends of adolescents with type 1 DM, is associated with improved DM knowledge and social support of DM care, as well as parent report of decreased conflict at home.[118]

In the general population, intensive multisystemic therapy (MST) has been applied primarily to adolescents with antisocial behaviors and criminal histories.[119] MST expands upon previous systems-based approaches by considering multiple systems, including family (both immediate and extended), peers, school, and community, as important areas to target. MST does not follow a session by session protocol and is difficult to operationalize, but often includes techniques from CBT, parent training, and behavioral family systems therapy.[119,120] A multisystemic, home-based intervention with 8–17-year-olds targeting both peer and family support has been described by Pendley et al, with preliminary findings suggesting that peer participation in the intervention is associated with improved metabolic control.[121] A recent study indicates that MST targeting chronically poorly controlled adolescents with type 1 DM has been associated with reduced diabetes-related stress, improved regimen adherence, and decreased inpatient admissions and care costs associated with diabetes.[122]

Conclusions

Considerable research has shown that psychosocial factors play a crucial role in the management of DM in both children and adults. The research evidence indicates that individuals with DM are at increased risk for psychosocial difficulties and psychiatric disorders, particularly depression, anxiety disorders, and eating disorders. When present, these disorders appear to be associated with problems with diabetes management and increased likelihood for poor glycemic control, diabetes-related health complications, and hospitalizations. Studies have demonstrated that family factors are associated with regimen adherence and glycemic control, with the best outcomes attained for individuals whose families communicate well, provide support, and are appropriately involved in diabetes care. Research has also shown the efficacy of several types of psychosocial therapies that can improve regimen adherence and glycemic control, as well as psychosocial functioning and quality of life. However, more research is needed to develop psychosocial intervention programs for specific patient populations with various psychiatric disorders, and to demonstrate the cost-effectiveness of these approaches.

References

1. Delamater AM, Jacobson AM, Anderson B. Psychosocial therapies in diabetes. Report of the psychosocial therapies working group. Diabetes Care 2001; 24: 1286–92.
2. DiMatteo MR, Lepper HS, Croghan TW. Depression is a risk factor for noncompliance with medical treatment: meta-analysis of the effects of anxiety and depression on patient adherence. Arch Intern Med 2000; 160: 2101–7.
3. Lustman PJ, Anderson RJ, Freedland KE et al. Depression and poor glycemic control: a meta-analytic review of the literature. Diabetes Care 2000; 23: 934–42.
4. de Groot M, Anderson R, Freedland KE et al. Association of depression and diabetes complications: a meta-analysis. Psychosom Med 2001; 63: 619–30.
5. Anderson RJ, Freedland KE, Clouse RE et al. The prevalence of comorbid depression in adults with diabetes: a meta-analysis. Diabetes Care 2001; 24: 1069–78.
6. Chambless DL, Baker MJ, Baucom DH et al. Update on empirically validated therapies, II. Clin Psychologist 1998; 51: 3–16.
7. Harris MD. Psychosocial aspects of diabetes with an emphasis on depression. Curr Diab Rep 2003; 2: 49–55.
8. Fisher L, Chesla CA, Mullan JT et al. Contributors to depression in Latino and European-American patients with type 2 diabetes. Diabetes Care 2001; 24: 1751–7.
9. Lustman PJ, Griffith LS, Freedland KE et al. Cognitive behavior therapy for depression in type 2 diabetes mellitus: a randomized, controlled trial. Ann Intern Med 1998; 129: 613–21.
10. Musselman DL, Betan E, Larsen H et al. Relationship of depression to diabetes type 1 and 2: epidemiology, biology, and treatment. Biol Psychiatry 2003; 54: 317–29.
11. Lustman PJ, Freedland KE, Griffith LS et al. Predicting response to cognitive behavior therapy of depression in type 2 diabetes. Gen Hosp Psychiatry 1998; 20: 302–6.
12. Cornes CL, Frank E. Interpersonal psychotherapy for depression. Clin Psychologist 1994; 47: 9–10.
13. Rubin RR, Peyrot M. Psychological issues and treatments for people with diabetes. J Clin Psychol 2001; 57: 457–78.
14. Hegel M, Arean P. Problem Solving Treatment for Primary Care (PST-PC): A Treatment Manual for Depression. Darthmouth: NH Project IMPACT, 2003.
15. Katon WJ, Von Korff M, Lin EH et al. The Pathways Study: a randomized trial of collaborative care in patients with diabetes and depression. Arch Gen Psychiatry 2004; 61: 1042–9.
16. Wiliams JW, Katon W, Lin EH et al. The effectiveness of depression care management on diabetes-related outcomes in older patients. Ann Intern Med 2004; 140: 1015–24.

17. Lustman PJ, Freedland KE, Griffith LS et al. Fluoxetine for depression in diabetes: a randomized double-blind placebo-controlled trial. Diabetes Care 2000; 23: 618–23.

18. Lustman PJ, Griffith LS, Clouse RE et al. Effects of nortriptyline on depression and glycemic control in diabetes: results of a double-blind, placebo-controlled trial. Psychosom Med 1997; 59: 241–50.

19. Keller MB, McCullough JP, Klein DN et al. A comparison of nefazodone, the cognitive-behavioral analysis system of psychotherapy, and their combination for the treatment of chronic depression. N Engl J Med 2000; 342: 1462–70.

20. Lustman PJ, Griffith LS, Freedland KE et al. The course of major depression in diabetes. Gen Hosp Psychiatry 1997; 19: 138–43.

21. Piette JD, Richardson C, Valenstein M. Addressing the needs of patients with multiple chronic illnesses: the case of diabetes and depression. Am J Manag Care 2004; 10: 152–62.

22. Surwit RS, Schneider MS. Role of stress in the etiology and treatment of diabetes mellitus. Psychosom Med 1993; 55: 380–93.

23. Aikens JE, Kiolbasa TA, Sobel R. Psychological predictors of glycemic change with relaxation training in non-insulin-dependent diabetes mellitus. Psychother Psychosom 1997; 66: 302–6.

24. Jablon SL, Naliboff BD, Gilmore SL et al. Effects of relaxation training on glucose tolerance and diabetic control in type II diabetes. Appl Psychophysiol Biofeedback 1997; 22: 155–69.

25. Lane JD, McCaskill CC, Ross SL et al. Relaxation training for NIDDM. Predicting who may benefit. Diabetes Care 1993; 16: 1087–94.

26. McGinnis RA, McGrady A, Cox S et al. Biofeedback-assisted relaxation in type 2 diabetes. Diabetes Care 2005; 28: 2145–9.

27. McGrady A, Horner J. Role of mood in outcome of biofeedback assisted relaxation therapy in insulin dependent diabetes mellitus. Appl Psychophysiol Biofeedback 1999; 24: 79–88.

28. Surwit RS, van Tilburg MA, Zucker N et al. Stress management improves long-term glycemic control in type 2 diabetes. Diabetes Care 2002; 25: 30–4.

29. Tsujiuchi T, Kumano H, Yoshiuchi K et al. The Effect of Qi-gong relaxation exercise on the control of type 2 diabetes mellitus: a randomized controlled trial. Diabetes Care 2002; 25: 241–2.

30. Karlsen B, Idsoe T, Dirdal I et al. Effects of a group based counselling programme on diabetes-related stress, coping, psychological well-being, and metabolic control in adults with type 1 or type 2 diabetes. Patient Educ Couns 2004; 53: 299–308.

31. Henry JL, Wilson PH, Bruce DG et al. Cognitive-behavioural stress management for patients with non-insulin dependent diabetes mellitus. Psychol Health Med 1997; 2: 109–18.

32. Spiess K, Sachs G, Pietschmann P et al. A program to reduce onset distress in unselected type 1 diabetic patients: effects on psychological variables and metabolic control. Eur J Endocrinol 1995; 132: 580–6.

33. Zettler A, Duran G, Waadt S et al. Coping with fear of long-term complications in diabetes mellitus: a model clinical program. Psychother Psychosom 1995; 64: 178–84.

34. Costea M, Ionescu-Tirgoviste C, Cheta D et al. Fear of hypoglycemia in type 1 (insulin-dependent) diabetic patients. Rom J Intern Med 1993; 31: 291–5.

35. Mollema ED, Snoek FJ, Ader HJ et al. Insulin-treated diabetes patients with fear of self-injecting or fear of self-testing: psychological comorbidity and general well-being. J Psychosom Res 2001; 51: 665–72.

36. Bienvenu OJ, Eaton WW. The epidemiology of blood-injection-injury phobia. Psychol Med 1998; 28: 1129–36.

37. Zambanini A, Newson RB, Maisey M et al. Injection related anxiety in insulin-treated diabetes. Diabetes Res Clin Pract 1999; 46: 239–46.

38. Boyle S, Allan C, Millar K. Cognitive-behavioural interventions in a patient with an anxiety disorder related to diabetes. Behav Res Ther 2004; 42: 357–66.

39. Green L, Feher M, Catalan J. Fears and phobias in people with diabetes. Diabetes Metab Res Rev 2000; 16: 287–93.

40. Polonsky WH, Davis CL, Jacobson AM et al. Correlates of hypoglycemic fear in type 1 and type 2 diabetes mellitus. Health Psychol 1992; 11: 199–202.

41. Steel JM, Masterson G, Patrick AW et al. Hyperventilation or hypoglycaemia? Diabet Med 1989; 6: 820–1.

42. Herpertz S, Wagener R, Albus C et al. Diabetes mellitus and eating disorders: a multicenter study on the comorbidity of the two diseases. J Psychosom Res 1998; 44: 503–15.

43. Jones JM, Lawson M, Daneman D, Olmsted MP, Rodin G. Eating disorders in adolescent females with and without type 1 diabetes: cross-sectional study. BMJ 2000; 320: 1563–6.

44. Hoffman RP. Eating disorders in adolescents with type 1 diabetes. A closer look at a complicated condition. Postgrad Med 2001; 109: 67–74.

45. Fairburn CG, Jones R, Peveler RC et al. Psychotherapy and bulimia nervosa. Longer-term effects of interpersonal psychotherapy, behavior therapy, and cognitive behavior therapy. Arch Gen Psychiatry 1993; 50: 419–28.

46. Rosen DS. Eating disorders in children and young adolescents: etiology, classification, clinical features, and treatment. Adolesc Med 2003; 14: 677–89.

47. Biggs MM, Basco MR, Patterson G et al. Insulin withholding for weight control in women with diabetes. Diabetes Care 1994; 17: 1186–9.

48. Polonsky WH, Anderson BJ, Lohrer PA et al. Insulin omission in women with IDDM. Diabetes Care 1994; 17: 1178–85.

49. Kelly SD, Howe CJ, Hendler JP et al. Disordered eating behaviors in youth with type 1 diabetes. Diabetes Educ 2005; 31: 572–83.

50. Daneman D, Olmsted M, Rydall A et al. Eating disorders in young women with type 1 diabetes. Prevalence, problems and prevention. Horm Res 1998; 50(Suppl 1): 79–86.

51. Malone GL, Armstrong BK. Treatment of anorexia nervosa in a young adult patient with diabetes mellitus. J Nerv Ment Dis 1985; 173: 509–11.

52. Peveler RC, Fairburn CG. Anorexia nervosa in association with diabetes mellitus – a cognitive-behavioural approach to treatment. Behav Res Ther 1989; 27: 95–9.

53. Olmsted MP, Daneman D, Rydall AC, Lawson ML, Rodin G. The effects of psychoeducation on disturbed eating attitudes and behavior in young women with type 1 diabetes mellitus. Int J Eat Disord 2002; 32: 230–9.

54. Alloway SC, Toth EL, McCargar LJ. Effectiveness of a group psychoeducation program for the treatment of subclinical disordered eating in women with type 1 diabetes. Can J Diet Pract Res 2001; 62: 188–92.

55. van der Ven N. Psychosocial group interventions in diabetes care. Diabetes Spectrum 2003; 16: 88–95.

56. Takii M, Uchigata Y, Komaki G et al. An integrated inpatient therapy for type 1 diabetic females with bulimia nervosa: a 3-year follow-up study. J Psychosom Res 2003; 55: 349–56.

57. Kenardy J, Mensch M, Bowen K, Green B, Walton J. Group therapy for binge eating in Type 2 diabetes: a randomized trial. Diabet Med 2002; 19: 234–9.

58. Dantzer C, Swedenson J, Maurice-Tison S et al. Anxiety and depression in juvenile diabetes: a critical review. Clin Psychol Rev 2003; 23: 787–800.

59. Kovacs M, Obrsoky DS, Goldston D et al. Major depressive disorder in youths with IDDM. Diabetes Care 1997; 20: 45–51.

60. Grey M, Cameron ME, Lipman TH et al. Psychosocial status of children with diabetes in the first two years after diagnosis. Diabetes Care 1995; 18: 1330–6.

61. Blanz BJ, Rensch-Reimann BS, Fritz-Sigmund DI et al. IDDM is a risk factor for adolescent psychiatric disorders. Diabetes Care 1993; 16: 1579–87.

62. Kovacs M, Goldston D, Obrsoky DS et al. Psychiatric disorders in youths with IDDM: rates and risk factors. Diabetes Care 1997; 20: 36–44.

63. Grey M, Whittemore R, Tamborlane W. Depression and type 1 diabetes in children: natural history and correlates. J Psychosom Res 2002; 53: 907–11.

64. Goldston DB, Kovacs M, Ho VY et al. Suicidal ideation and suicide attempts among youths with insulin-dependent diabetes mellitus. J Am Acad Child Adolesc Psychiatry 1994; 33: 240–6.

65. Jacobson AM, Hauser ST, Willet J et al. Psychological adjustment to IDDM: 10-year follow up of an onset cohort of child and adolescent patients. Diabetes Care 1997; 20: 811–8.

66. Vila G, Nollet-Clemenson C, Vera M et al. Prevalence of DSM-IV disorders in children and adolescents with asthma versus diabetes. Can J Psychiatry 1999; 44: 562–9.

67. Gold MA, Gladstein J. Substance abuse among adolescents with diabetes mellitus: preliminary findings. J Adolesc Health 1993; 14: 80–4.

68. Glasgow AM, Tynan D, Schwartz R et al. Alcohol and drug use in teenagers with diabetes mellitus. J Adolesc Health 1991; 12: 11–14.

69. Frey MA, Guthrie B, Loveland-Cherry C, Park PS, Foster CM. Risky behaviors and risk in adolescents with IDDM. J Adolesc Health 1997; 20: 38–45.

70. Kovacs M, Ho V, Pollock MH. Criterion and predictive validity of the diagnosis of adjustment disorder: A prospective study of youths with new-onset insulin-dependent diabetes mellitus. Am J Psychiatry 1995; 152: 523–8.

71. Jacobson AM, Hauser ST, Lavori P et al. Family environment and glycemic control: a four-year prospective study of children and adolescents with insulin-dependent diabetes mellitus. Psychosom Med 1994; 56: 401–9.

72. Grey M, Cameron M, Lipman T, Thurber F. Psychosocial status of children with diabetes in the first 2 years after diagnosis. Diabetes Care 1995; 18: 1330–6.

73. Daviss W, Burleson MD, Coon H et al. Predicting diabetic control from competence, adherence, adjustment and psychopathology. J Am Acad Child Adolesc Psychiatry 1995; 34: 1629–36.

74. Nordfeldt S, Ludvigsson J. Fear and other disturbances of severe hypoglycaemia in children and adolescents with type 1 diabetes mellitus. J Pediatr Endocrinol Metab 2005; 18: 83–91.

75. Dammacco F, Torelli C, Frezza E, Piccinno E, Tansella F. Problems of hypoglycemia arising in children and adolescents with insulin-dependent diabetes mellitus. The Diabetes Study Group of The Italian Society of Pediatric Endocrinology & Diabetes. J Pediatr Endocrinol Metab 1998; 11(Suppl 1): 167–76.

76. Green LB, Wysocki T, Reineck BM. Fear of hypoglycemia in children and adolescents with diabetes. J Pediatr Psychol 1990; 15: 633–41.

77. Davidson M, Penney ED, Muller B et al. Stressors and self-care challenges faced by adolescents living with type 1 diabetes. Appl Nurs Res 2004; 17: 72–80.

78. Northam EA, Matthews LK, Anderson PJ, Cameron FJ, Werther GA. Psychiatric morbidity and health outcomes in type 1 diabetes – perspectives from a prospective longitudinal study. Diabet Med 2004; 22: 152–7.

79. Stewart S, Rao U, Emslie G et al. Depressive symptoms predict hospitalizations for adolescents with type 1 diabetes. Pediatrics 2005; 115: 1315–19.

80. Kovacs M, Mukerji P, Iyengar S et al. Psychiatric disorder and metabolic control among youths with IDDM. A longitudinal study. Diabetes Care 1996; 19: 318–23.

81. Garrison M, Katon W, Richardson L. The impact of psychiatric comorbidities on readmissions for diabetes in youth. Diabetes Care 2005; 28: 2150–4.

82. Bryden KS, Peveler RC, Stein A et al. Clinical and psychological course of diabetes from adolescents to young adulthood. Diabetes Care 2001; 24: 1536–40.

83. Lernmark B, Persson B, Fisher L, Rydelius PA. Symptoms of depression are important to psychological adaptation and metabolic control in children with diabetes mellitus. Diabet Med 1999; 16: 14–22.

84. Leonard B, Jang Y, Savik K, Plumbo PM, Christensen R. Psychosocial factors associated with levels of metabolic control in youth with type 1 diabetes. J Pediatr Nurs 2002; 17: 28–37.

85. Dumont RH, Jacobson AM, Cole C et al. Psychosocial predictors of acute complications of diabetes in youth. Diabet Med 1995; 12: 612–18.

86. Liss DS, Waller DA, Kennard BD et al. Psychiatric illness and family support in children and adolescents with diabetic ketoacidosis: a controlled study. J Am Acad Child Adolesc Psychiatry 1998; 37: 536–44.

87. Anderson BJ, Vangsness AL, Connell A et al. Family conflict, adherence, and glycaemic control in youth with short duration Type 1 diabetes. Diabet Med 2002; 19: 635–42.

88. Laffel LM, Connell A, Vangsness L et al. General quality of life in youth with type 1 diabetes: relationship to patient management and diabetes-specific family conflict. Diabetes Care 2003; 26: 3067–73.

89. Davis CL, Delamater AM, Shaw KH et al. Parenting styles, regimen adherence, and glycemic control in 4- to 10-year-old children with diabetes. J Pediatr Psychol 2001; 26: 123–9.

90. Worrall-Davis A, Holland P, Berg I, Goodyer I. The effects of adverse life events on glycaemic control in children with insulin dependent diabetes mellitus. Eur Child Adolesc Psychiatry 1999; 8: 11–16.

91. Boland EA, Grey M. Coping strategies of school-age children with diabetes mellitus. Diabetes Educ 1996; 22: 592–7.

92. Grey M, Lipman T, Cameron ME et al. Coping behaviors at diagnosis and in adjustment one year later in children with diabetes. Nurs Res 1997; 46: 312–17.

93. Delamater AM, Kurtz SM, Bubb J, White NH, Santiago JV. Stress and coping in relation to metabolic control of adolescents with type I diabetes. J Dev Behav Pediatr 1987; 8: 136–40.

94. Hampson SE, Skinner TC, Hart J et al. Behavioral interventions for adolescents with type 1 diabetes. How effective are they? Diabetes Care 2000; 23: 1416–22.

95. Allen KD, Evans JH. Exposure-based treatment to control excessive blood glucose monitoring. J Appl Behav Anal 2001; 34: 497–500.

96. Moore KE, Geffken GR, Royal GP. Behavioral intervention to reduce child distress during self-injection. Clin Pediatr 1995; 34: 530–4.

97. Boardway RH, Delamater AM, Tomakowsky J, Gutai JP. Stress management training for adolescents with diabetes. J Pediatr Psychol 1993; 18: 29–45.

98. Hains AA, Davies WH, Parton E, Totka J, Amoroso-Camarata J. A stress management intervention for adolescents with type 1 diabetes. Diabetes Educ 2000; 26: 417–23.

99. Hains AA, Davies WH, Parton E, Silverman AH. Brief report: a cognitive behavioral intervention for distressed adolescents with type I diabetes. J Pediatr Psychol 2001; 26: 61–6.

100. Bendez FJ, Belendez M. Effects of a behavioral intervention on treatment adherence and stress management in adolescents with IDDM. Diabetes Care 1997; 20: 1370–5.

101. Grey M, Boland EA, Davidson M et al. Short-term effects of coping skills training as adjunct to intensive therapy in adolescents. Diabetes Care 1998; 21: 902–8.

102. Boland EA, Grey M, Oesterle Al, Fredrickson L, Tamborlane WV. Continuous subcutaneous insulin infusion. A new way to lower risk of severe hypoglycemia, improve metabolic control, and enhance coping in adolescents with type 1 diabetes. Diabetes Care 1999; 22: 1779–84.

103. Grey M, Boland EA, Davidson M, Li J, Tamborlane W. Coping skills training for youth with diabetes mellitus has long-lasting effects on metabolic control and quality of life. J Pediatr 2000; 137: 107–13.

104. Cook S, Herold K, Edidin DV, Briars R. Increasing problem solving in adolescents with type 1 diabetes: the choices diabetes program. Diabetes Educ 2002; 28: 115–24.

105. Auslander WF, Bubb J, Rogge M et al. Family stress and resources: potential areas of intervention in children recently diagnosed with diabetes. Health Soc Work 1993; 18: 101–13.

106. Delamater AM, Bubb J, Davis SG et al. Randomized, prospective study of self-management training with newly diagnosed diabetic children. Diabetes Care 1990; 13: 492–8.

107. Svoren B, Butler D, Levine BS, Anderson BJ, Laffel LM. Reducing acute adverse outcomes in youths with type 1 diabetes: A randomized, controlled trial. Pediatrics 2003; 112: 914–22.

108. Anderson BJ, Brackett J, Ho J, Laffel LM. An office-based intervention to maintain parent–adolescent teamwork in diabetes management. Impact on parental involvement, family conflict, and subsequent glycemic control. Diabetes Care 1999; 22: 713–21.

109. Laffel LM, Vangsness L, Connell A et al. Impact of ambulatory, family-focused teamwork intervention on glycemic control in youth with type 1 diabetes. J Pediatr 2003; 142: 409–16.

110. Delamater AM, Smith JA, Bubb J et al. Family-based behavior therapy for diabetic adolescents. In: Johnson JH, Johnson SB, eds. Advances in Child Health Psychology. Gainesville, FL: University of Florida Press, 1991: 293–306.

111. Satin W, La Greca AM, Zigo MA, Skyler JS. Diabetes in adolescence: effects of multifamily group intervention and parent simulation of diabetes. J Pediatr Psychol 1989; 14: 259–75.

112. Wysocki T, Harris MA, Greco P et al. Social validity of support group and behavior therapy interventions for families of adolescents with insulin-dependent diabetes mellitus. J Pediatr Psychol 1997; 22: 635–49.

113. Wysocki T, Harris MA, Greco P et al. Randomized, controlled trial of behavior therapy for families of adolescents with insulin-dependent diabetes mellitus. J Pediatr Psychol 2000; 25: 23–33.
114. Wysocki T, Harris MA, Buckloh LM et al. Effects of behavioral family systems therapy for diabetes on adolescents' family relationships, treatment adherence, and metabolic control. J Pediatr Psychol 2006; Advanced Access http: //jpepsy.oxfordjournals.org/cgi/content/abstract/jsj098v1.
115. Robin A, Foster S. Negotiating Parent–Adolescent Conflict: A Behavioral-Family Systems Approach. New York, NY: The Guilford Press, 1989.
116. Jacobson AM, Hauser ST, Lavori P et al. Adherence among children and adolescents with insulin-dependent diabetes mellitus over a four-year longitudinal follow-up: I. The influence of patient coping and adjustment. J Pediatr Psychol 1990; 15: 511–26.
117. Johnson SB, Kelly M, Henretta JC et al. A longitudinal analysis of adherence and health status in childhood diabetes. J Pediatr Psychol 1992; 17: 537–53.
118. Greco P, Pendley JS, McDonell K et al. A peer group intervention for adolescents with type 1 diabetes and their best friends. J Pediatr Psychol 2001; 26: 485–90.
119. Kazdin AE, Weisz JR. Identifying and developing empirically supported child and adolescent treatments. J Consult Clin Psychol 1998; 66: 19–36.
120. Ellis DA, Frey MA, Naar-King S et al. The effects of multisystemic therapy on diabetes stress among adolescents with chronically poorly controlled type 1 diabetes: findings from a randomized, controlled trial. Pediatrics 2005; 116: 826–32.
121. Pendley JS, Kasmen LJ, Miller DL et al. Peer and family support in children and adolescents with type 1 diabetes. J Pediatr Psychol 2002; 27: 429–38.
122. Ellis DA, Naar-King S, Frey M et al. Multisystemic treatment of poorly controlled type 1 diabetes: effects on medical resource utilization. J Pediatr Psychol 2005; 30: 656–66.

Chapter 13

Collaborative care to improve treatment of co-occurring diabetes mellitus and psychiatric disorders

Maria D Llorente and Jesica Soto

Introduction

Psychiatric disorders are prevalent and associated with several medical comorbidities. Health care disparities have recently been attributed to the presence of having a psychiatric disorder. A growing body of evidence has suggested that integrated or collaborative care models of primary care and mental health services delivery may lead to improved medical and psychiatric outcomes among patients with psychiatric disorders. Whereas models have been described to address anxiety disorders (especially panic disorder) and at-risk alcohol use and abuse, this chapter will focus on several models of health services delivery that address psychiatric outcomes in the primary care setting, with particular focus on depressive disorders and diabetes mellitus (DM) due to their frequent co-occurrence.

Health care disparities and psychiatric disorders

Whereas a significant body of literature exists detailing racial and ethnic disparities in health care,[1] a growing evidence base has begun to describe health care disparities associated with having a psychiatric disorder. Psychiatric disorders are quite prevalent and are expected to account for 15% of disability adjusted life-years worldwide by 2020.[2] In fact, 5 of the top 10 causes of disability in the world are mental disorders (major depression, schizophrenia, bipolar disorder, alcohol abuse, and obsessive-compulsive disorder). In the USA, psychiatric disorders affect 20–30% of the population.[3,4] Individuals with psychiatric disorders have higher mortality rates at earlier ages,[5-8] lower quality of care for co-occurring medical illnesses,[9-15] and higher health care costs[16,17] than patients without mental illness. Furthermore, many of these studies were conducted with patients in the Department of Veterans Affairs Veterans Health Administration (VHA) where there is an emphasis on medical care for patients with psychiatric disorders. It is likely that these disparities may be larger in diverse clinical systems, particularly those with limited access to primary care services. Additionally, because there is an increased prevalence of several chronic medical conditions (i.e. diabetes, cardiovascular disease) among patients with psychiatric illness, this represents a significant public health issue.

Identification of the various factors that could explain these disparities is important in order to develop appropriate intervention strategies. Medical outcomes may vary based on patient variables such as psychiatric diagnosis, communication and access barriers, and adherence issues. For example, patients with certain psychiatric conditions, notably substance use disorders, are known to underutilize preventive medical services.[15,18] This suggests that addressing medical problems might best occur within the setting of a specialty substance abuse treatment program. Similarly, provider factors, including lack of training in ambulatory psychiatry diagnosis and management, time constraints, and bias against 'difficult' patients, can adversely impact delivery of services. This is supported by data indicating that patients with personality disorders have more pronounced disparities,[15] and suggests that integration of mental health and primary care may address these issues. Lastly, systems issues, notably, institutional emphasis on enhanced access and care for patients with mental health problems, may ultimately prove to be a significant factor. Other patient-, provider- and systems-specific factors may yet be described with further investigation.

There are several possible descriptions of the relationship that can occur between mental health (MH) and primary care (PC) providers. At one end of this continuum, the MH and PC providers may function autonomously, with no communication or collaboration. A second type of relationship occurs when the PC provider may identify an MH problem, and then refer the patient, essentially 'handing off' the responsibility of patient care over to the MH consultant. There may be initial contact, with the PC provider explaining the reason for the referral, and the MH provider responding with findings, diagnosis, and an initial plan of care, but little collaboration or future communications occur thereafter. A third type of relationship involves a closer consultative relationship in which there is increased communication and collaboration between the MH and PC providers. They may share a common medical chart, be co-located, or have periodic joint team meetings to discuss patient cases. At the other end of the continuum is the fourth type of relationship, joint care. MH and PC providers are typically co-located in the same clinical setting. They frequently communicate, often in person, and share responsibility for the management of the psychiatric disorder. It is hypothesized that this type of care is likely to lead to improved MH and medical outcomes. Interestingly, there are two potential collaborative arrangements. An MH care provider may be co-located in a PC setting, seeing patients for psychosocial problems, and available for immediate consultation to the PC clinicians. Alternatively, a PC provider could be co-located in an MH care setting, seeing patients for primary care issues, and available for immediate consultation to the MH clinicians.

Integration of mental health in primary care

Because most persons seeking care for psychiatric disorders first go to their primary care provider, several efforts have tried to improve the identification and treatment of psychiatric illness in primary care. Much of this work has been done using depression as the target psychiatric illness. Traditional methods have included enhanced training of PC clinicians through providing practice guidelines, lectures, and direct-to-physician conferences.[19] These efforts fail to change clinical practice, unless additional incentives are provided. Other strategies have been to introduce computer-driven decision support,[20] automated scheduling of follow-up appointments,[21] enhanced mental health screening, extensive physician feedback, and monitoring of clinical response with severity measures.[22,23] Enhancements include selecting mental health clinics with services tailored to specific patient populations, providing transportation and third-party payment coverage, and minimizing the time from referral to visit with the specialty mental health provider.[24,25] Consistent improvements in psychiatric outcomes, however, have not been seen.

More recently, several models have been developed to improve mental health services in primary care and typically call for either collaboration between mental health and primary care providers or for the integration of mental health providers into primary care settings.[24] Potential advantages of integrated, collaborative care include:

- increased recognition of mental illness
- decreased stigma
- increased access to MH services
- fewer no-show appointments
- avoidance of the mind–body split
- improved communication between MH and PC providers
- enhanced continuity of care
- opportunities for professional development on the part of the providers.

Possible disadvantages of integrated care may include:

- focus on short-term treatment
- specialized services (e.g. group therapy) not available
- financial/third party payment issues
- privacy of medical records.

An added consideration is that both PC and MH providers need to feel comfortable working side-by-side, being readily available for consultation to each other, and be able and willing to share responsibility for patient care issues.

Katon et al[26] found that a collaborative care model increased antidepressant medication adherence and symptom improvements in patients with major depression, but it did not appear to affect outcomes for patients with minor depression (especially older patients). A limitation of this model was the reliance on psychiatrists as the mental health care provider. In a subsequent study, use of non-psychiatrists and a structured depression treatment program that included both behavioral treatment and medication adherence counseling, patients with major depression showed improvement on all outcomes measured, including medication adherence, satisfaction, symptom reduction, and health care visits[27] in a mixed-age group.

As previously noted, many of these studies have chosen depression as the prototype psychiatric illness for a variety of reasons. First, depression is a highly prevalent disease,[2-4] associated with a great deal of morbidity and disability,[6-8,28] if left untreated. Secondly, there is a solid evidence base in support of routine screening for depression,[24,29] with several reliable case-finding instruments available.[29,30] Thirdly, depression is one of the most treatable mental disorders, with clear guideline-based recommendations for adequate treatment.[24,29] Lastly, the majority of patients with depressive disorders are seen and treated by primary care providers.[3]

Similarly, while several medical conditions are prevalent among patients with psychiatric disorders, DM is a particularly useful medical condition to study for several reasons. First, diabetes frequently co-occurs with several psychiatric disorders. Secondly, the evidence base for DM management is strong. Lastly, performance measures with objective outcome targets for recommended care exist and are easy to monitor and compare. Most collaborative care models studied to date have included patients with a specific psychiatric disorder (depression) and various medical comorbidities, and have been primarily conducted with an older adult population.

Unified Psychogeriatric Biopsychosocial Evaluation And Treatment (UPBEAT)

UPBEAT was a multisite randomized national clinical demonstration project comparing a collaborative care intervention with usual care. This study aimed to examine mental and physical health outcomes, health care utilization and cost, and patient satisfaction in a mental health care coordination model targeting medically ill older veterans with unrecognized symptoms of depression, anxiety, and/or alcohol abuse. A clinical care coordination model was adopted to provide early psychiatric intervention in order to treat unrecognized mental health problems, decrease hospitalizations, improve quality of life, and allow the veteran to remain independent as long as possible.

The study intervention incorporated an in-depth structured diagnostic assessment, assignment to a care coordinator (nurse, social worker, or psychologist), collaboration between PC and MH clinicians, inclusion of patient preferences in an individualized multidisciplinary care plan, proactive follow-up, and outcomes monitoring by the care coordinator. The treatment plan addressed medical, psychiatric, and psychosocial issues, and was updated on a regular basis.

Patients were recruited from 9 VHA medical centers in three geographic regions (California, Florida, and Northeastern USA). A total of 1687 patients met target diagnostic criteria and were randomized to receive the collaborative intervention or usual care. Patients were followed for 12 months. The mean age of the sample was 69.4 years and 26% of the sample were ethnic or racial minority elderly.

The UPBEAT patients had statistically significant improvement ($p>0.05$) in baseline physical and mental roles, mental health, and bodily pain at 12-month follow-up.[31,32] The relative improvement, compared with the usual care group, though, was less than expected due to substantial improvement in the usual care patients. Among the 1687 patients enrolled, inpatient days decreased more for the interventional arm (–8.7 days/patient/year) than for usual care (–4.8 days/patient/year); this difference was statistically significant ($p=0.015$). While UPBEAT also increased outpatient costs by $1171 per patient, there was still an overall cost savings of $1856 per patient, achieving net health care cost savings of over $3 million nationally in the first year of the intervention. Eighty percent of UPBEAT patients reported high degrees of satisfaction with care, compared with only 45% of nationally surveyed veterans.

Additionally, as part of a local pilot quality improvement project, 56 patients with diabetes and significant depressive symptoms were identified at the Miami UPBEAT site. At baseline, compliance with three clinical guideline outcomes in diabetes was measured: (1) glycosylated $HbA_{1c}<9\%$; (2) annual foot sensory examination; and (3) annual retinal examination. All veterans had comparable baseline levels of compliance that were statistically lower than national averages and benchmarks. Half the subjects ($n=28$) were randomized to usual care and half ($n=28$) were receiving a clinical care coordination (CCC) model of integrated mental health services for older veterans with comorbid chronic medical diseases. Only patients in the CCC group received the CCC intervention, consisting of assignment to a care coordinator (nurse), a multidisciplinary evaluation, and treatment plan development. At 3-month follow-up, compliance with the guideline outcomes had statistically improved in the CCC intervention group on all three measures. In particular, 92% of the patients in the interventional arm had improved glycemic control as measured by the HgA$_{1c}$ levels vs only 65% in the usual care group ($p > 0.05$).

Primary Care Research in Substance Abuse and Mental Health for the Elderly (PRISM-E)

The PRISM-E study was a multisite randomized trial comparing integrated and enhanced referral models of mental health care for older persons with depression, anxiety, and/or at-risk alcohol consumption.[33,34] The integrated model provided MH services in the primary care setting by a mental health provider. The enhanced referral model provided MH services in a specialty setting that was physically separate and designated as a mental health and/or substance abuse clinic. PRISM-E recognized that the term 'integration' is a complex construct and identified seven dimensions that reflect the degree of integratedness of MH services in primary care (Table 13.1). The specific model used at each site had to be consistent with these seven dimensions, but was site-specific.

Participants were recruited from five VA medical centers, three community health centers, and two outpatient hospital networks. More than 24 000 primary care patients aged ≥ 65 years were screened for the presence of a mental health disorder or at-risk drinking, and of these, more than 2000 completed baseline assessments and met criteria for the target diagnoses. The mean age of the sample was 73.5 years, with a significant proportion of ethnic minority elderly (48% of the total sample). Two-thirds had a primary diagnosis of depression, and on average, had 4.7 chronic medical conditions. Approximately 26% of the sample had diabetes. Patients were followed for a minimum of 6 months.

Integrated care was associated with higher rates of engagement in MH services (71% vs 49% in the enhanced referral model [OR = 2.57; 95% CI 2.14–3.08]), and more MH visits per patient (mean = 3.04), compared with enhanced referral (mean = 1.91) ($p < 0.001$). For all conditions, greater engagement was associated with closer proximity of MH services to primary care.

Table 13.1 Dimensions of integration of mental health (MH) in primary care (PC)

Dimension	Conceptual framework
Responsibility	Extent to which the PC and MH share responsibility for MH care within the PC setting (vs 'handing over' responsibility to a specialty MH provider in less-integrated models)
Array of MH services	More highly integrated models provide a broader array of MH services within the PC setting, making it less necessary to refer patients to other sources to obtain these services
Provider expertise	More highly integrated models have a broader array of MH expertise within the PC settting or closely available to the PC setting
Communication	Extent to which MH and PC providers share information and communicate (more integrated have greater frequency and intensity and are more likely to communicate verbally and face-to-face)
Organizational structure	Extent to which PC and MH providers share organizational systems such as leadership, quality, management, performance monitoring, incentivizing arrangements, data systems, and billing systems
Physical proximity	More highly integrated models have fewer geographical barriers to MH care in terms of: (1) distance separating MH and PC setting; (2) need for transportation to two different settings; and (3) stigma because MH care is provided in a PC setting. The most integrated models have MH and PC services co-located in the same clinical area
Temporal proximity	More highly integrated models have little delay or time separation between the delivery of PC and MH services, leading to lower wait times, improved rates of initial and follow-up MH appointments, and higher rates of MH treatment engagement

PC = primary care; MH = mental health; PCP = primary care provider

Re-engineering Systems for the Primary Care Treatment of Depression (RESPECT-D)

This is a cluster randomized controlled comparison of an evidence-based depression care model with usual care in five health care organizations in the USA with 60 affiliated primary care practices.[35] A total of 400 patients were randomly assigned to the intervention or usual care arms, and were followed for 6 months. Mean age was 42 years, and approximately 80% were women.

The intervention consisted of a methodical approach to identify, diagnose, treat, and monitor response of depressive symptoms in primary care. The primary care provider retained responsibility for initiating treatment, but was supported by the efforts of a centrally based care manager (typically, a nurse with a mental health or primary care background). The care managers provided regular telephone and in-person support, psychoeducation, and encouraged self-management practices. A psychiatrist met with the care managers weekly to discuss new patients and was available for specialty consultation to the primary care providers.

At 6 months, 60% of the intervention patients had responded to treatment, with 37% remissions compared with 47% and 27% of those in usual care ($p < 0.02$ and $p < 0.014$, respectively). Additionally, 90% of the intervention group rated their care as good/excellent vs only 75% of the usual care group ($p < 0.0003$). The US Department of Defense, Deployment Health Clinical Center (DHCC) is in the process of implementing a modified model of this program to facilitate identification and treatment of returning veterans and their families.

Improving Mood – Promoting Access to Collaborative Treatment (IMPACT) for late-life depression

The IMPACT study was a multisite randomized controlled trial of a collaborative intervention program for enhanced depression treatment for late-life depression in primary care.[36-38] The study intervention incorporated evidence-based depression treatment (antidepressant medication, problem-solving psychotherapy, or both) with close collaboration between PC and MH clinicians. Follow-up and outcomes monitoring occurred regularly by a depression care manager (DCM), a nurse, or psychologist in the primary care clinic.

Patients were recruited from eight study organizations, consisting of 18 primary care clinics in five states. More than 32 000 patients were approached for screening. 1800 patients met target diagnostic criteria and were randomized to receive the collaborative intervention or usual care. While the intervention was for 12 months, patients were followed for up to 24 months. The mean age of the sample was

71.2 years, with, on average, 3.2 chronic medical conditions; 23% of the sample were ethnic or racial minority elderly. A subgroup analysis in 417 patients with diabetes was also completed.[37]

The IMPACT intervention included a 20-minute educational video-tape and a booklet about late-life depression. Patients were encouraged to have an initial visit with the DCM where their history and preferences regarding depression treatment (medications vs therapy) were obtained. The DCM also reviewed the educational materials. At a weekly team meeting, the DCM, the supervising psychiatrist, and a primary care physician discussed and developed recommendations regarding treatment. The DCM then worked with the patient and his/her primary care provider to establish the treatment plan, typically consisting of an initial choice of antidepressant (most commonly a selective serotonin receptor inhibitor [SSRI]) or a course of problem-solving treatment for primary care (PST-PC). The PST-PC is a brief, time-limited (6–8 sessions) structured psychotherapy for depression and was provided by the DCM.

If patients were already taking antidepressants, the dose could be increased, the medication changed, an augmenting agent added, and/or a trial of PST-PC could be started. The patient's PC provider retained responsibility for writing antidepressant prescriptions. The DCM could also encourage depression disease self-management techniques. The psychiatrist could see patients who were diagnostic challenges or who failed to respond to treatment. The Patient Health Questionnaire (PHQ-9)[30,39] was used to monitor treatment response as well as a web-based clinical information system.[40]

At 12 months, half of the IMPACT group reported at least a 50% reduction in depressive symptoms, vs only 19% of those in usual care.[36] Long-term follow-up indicated that, relative to usual care, IMPACT patients were more likely to continue antidepressant medication use and experience depression remission, had less severe depressive symptoms, and had better physical functioning, quality of life, self-efficacy, and satisfaction at both 18 and 24 months.[38] Among those patients with DM in the intervention group, depression symptoms responded ($p < 0.001$) and weekly exercise days increased ($p < 0.001$) relative to the usual care group. The response in depression was not associated with improved glycemic control or other diabetes self-management behaviors, however.[37] Whereas depression care was enhanced in this study, DM care was not, suggesting that collaborative care models must address both depression and DM self-management to achieve improved outcomes of both diseases.

Pathways Study

The Pathways Study is a multisite randomized controlled trial of a collaborative depression care program for mixed-age patients with DM.[41,42] The study intervention was similar to that used in the IMPACT study. Depression care enhancements included nurses with specialty MH training who collaborated with psychiatrists as consultants and primary care providers who initiated treatment. Patients were initially offered the choice of two evidence-based treatments: antidepressants or problem-solving therapy. Behavioral activation (exercise, goal-setting, healthy nutrition, problem-solving) was encouraged by the nurse care managers. Diabetes education was not a part of the program.

Patients were recruited from nine primary care clinics of a prepaid health plan enrolling approximately 500 000 persons in Washington state. Patients with DM were invited to participate and had to have a PHQ-9 score of ≥ 10. A total of 329 patients, randomized to receive either the intervention or usual care, were followed for up to 12 months. The mean age of the sample was 58.5 years, two-thirds were women, and 20% were from minority population groups. Patients predominantly had type 2 DM, with a mean HbA_{1c} of 8%, and had 1.5 diabetic complications.

Patients in the intervention arm had more adequate antidepressant treatment and less severe depression when compared with the usual care group. Overall, however, there were no between-group differences in diabetes self-management, and the intervention group exhibited lower adherence to oral hypoglycemic agents. These results again support the notion that both DM and depression need to be a simultaneous focus of treatment in collaborative care models in order to have beneficial outcomes in both disease states.

Prevention of Suicide in Primary Care Elderly: Collaborative Trial (PROSPECT)

The PROSPECT study is a multisite randomized controlled trial of a collaborative intervention program for late-life depression in primary care.[43,44] The study intervention was implemented by DCMs who used operationalized Agency for Health Care Policy and Research Guidelines.[29,45] The DCMs provided 'on-time and on-target' recommendations to primary care physicians, assisted patients with treatment adherence, monitored clinical symptoms, treatment response, and side effects, and assured follow-up care.

Patients were recruited from 20 primary care practices in three regions (New York City, Philadelphia, and Pittsburgh). Practices were paired by setting, academic affiliation, size, and minority distribution. Randomization was by practice to minimize potential contamination of usual care by the DCM. More than 16 000 patients were sampled, with 215 patients meeting target diagnostic criteria, and randomized to receive the collaborative intervention or usual care. Patients were followed for up to 18 months. The primary care physicians retained responsibility for the patient's MH clinical care. Initial recommendations included a trial of citalopram at a daily target dose of 30 mg. Patients who declined medication management were offered interpersonal psychotherapy by the DCM.

Results indicated that patients who received the PROSPECT intervention had less severe depressive symptoms and greater remission rates at 4, 8, and 12 months when compared with usual care. Remission occurred earlier for patients in the intervention practices. At 8 months, 43% of the PROSPECT participants had reached remission, vs 28% of patients receiving usual care. Of interest, those patients with higher levels of anxiety failed to respond to either PROSPECT intervention or usual care. Patients with comorbid anxiety and depression exhibit more severe symptoms overall, and generally have a longer course of illness, with poorer treatment response. Thus, patients with comorbid anxiety and depression may require a specialty referral to a psychiatrist.

Telemedicine And Care Coordination To Improve Care for Seniors (TACTICS)

TACTICS is a multidisciplinary clinical demonstration program that integrates a CCC model and telemedicine to implement evidence-based practices to enhance both diabetes and depression management simultaneously. Telemedicine has been shown to be cost-effective in a variety of health care settings.[46–48] Telemedicine encompasses a wide range of technologies, but the primary form of technology used by this program is an in-home messaging device that resembles a caller ID box and attaches to a standard telephone line (the Health Hero iCare Desktop and the Health Buddy appliance). The technology platform is based on several design features:

- flexibility, as key in targeting and addressing the needs of special populations
- simplicity, as essential to user compliance
- timeliness in data collection for disease self-management
- cost, as a critical issue in the practical application of disease management systems.[48]

Patients answer disease-specific questions each day regarding symptoms, medication compliance, and disease knowledge. Disease-specific patient education and feedback (in part, utilizing cognitive behavioral techniques) is then immediately provided by the device to the patient. The patient's answers are transmitted to a central, secure repository where the data are then made available to the CCC that same day (typically within a few hours) over the internet, through a secure website. Abnormal and blank responses are flagged. Responses from previous days are stored for reference. The responses are also color-coded to assist the CCC with prioritizing patient needs. The device facilitates disease self-management through a multi-tiered approach consisting of signs and symptoms reporting, targeted education around the targeted diseases (depression and diabetes), positive reinforcement for appropriate understanding of the disease, and adherence to recommended regimens, and also prompts the patient to action if indicated by daily signs and symptoms values.

Patients are recruited from the Miami VA Medical Center primary care and diabetes specialty care clinics and its nine outlying community-based outpatient clinics, and must have a clinical diagnosis of diabetes. Each patient is assigned to a care coordinator (MH nurse practitioner or registered dietician) who completes a structured psychiatric diagnostic assessment. Any patient meeting criteria for a psychiatric diagnosis is either referred to a psychiatrist affiliated with the program or, if already receiving mental health services, the results are discussed with the treating MH provider. Additionally, a diabetes knowledge assessment is performed, and any quality of care guideline diabetes measures (annual HbA_{1c}, foot sensory examination, retinal examination, blood pressure < 130/80 mmHg, control of dyslipidemias, use of ACE [angiotensin-converting enzyme] inhibitors, etc.) that are due or out of the desired range are addressed. Key components of the intervention are providing diabetes and depression disease self-management education and developing a nutritional plan that incorporates cultural and personal preferences. To date, 92 patients have enrolled in the program.

Preliminary results indicate that, at 6 months, Patient Health Questionnaire (PHQ-9) scores have decreased compared with baseline levels (10.7 vs 12.6, $p < 0.005$). At 12 months, several diabetes outcome measures have also improved, including blood pressure ($p < 0.003$), low-density lipoprotein (LDL) cholesterol ($p < 0.04$), and 100% of patients have a retinal and foot sensory examination. There are also trends toward improved HbA_{1c} (7.3% at baseline vs 6.8% at 12 months) and triglyceride levels (181 mg/dl at baseline vs 144 mg/dl at 12 months). Additionally, hospital admissions and emergency room visits were reduced by 67% and 60%, respectively. Total costs for admissions that did occur were reduced by 81% (from $56 794 at 6 months pre-enrollment to $10 906 in the 6 months after enrollment).

Regardless of the exact details of each program, several commonalities exist. Table 13.2[49] describes the personal characteristics and skill sets that make up the competencies that a mental health clinician working in a primary care setting should have. Additionally, general processes of care should follow those recommended by the MacArthur Initiative on Depression and Primary Care, listed in Table 13.3.[35,50]

Integration of primary care into mental health

For many patients with serious mental illness, specialty mental health settings are not only their initial entry into health care but are often their only contact with the health care system.[51] As a result, interest in providing primary care and medical preventive services in mental health settings may also be feasible,[52] although much less has been published in this area. One such model program has been described.[53] In this study, mental health assumed responsibility for the primary care needs of patients they were treating for serious mental illness. The primary care services were delivered in a clinic that was geographically contiguous to the mental health clinic. Clinical staffing included a primary care nurse practitioner (the main provider of medical services), a physician, and a nurse case manager. The case manager provided education, case management services, and collaborated with the mental health care providers. Communication occurred via telephone, email, and face-to-face meetings. A representative from this integrated team attended weekly team meetings with

Table 13.2   Competencies of mental health clinician working in
primary care

- Can come from a variety of disciplines (nursing, psychology, social work)
- Able to conduct mental health and substance abuse clinical assessments
- Able to provide the following types of clinical interventions:
  - Cognitive behavioral
  - Problem-solving
  - Psychoeducational
  - Group
- Basic knowledge of psychopharmacology
- Effective communication
- Able to work in a consultative capacity
- Flexible with team/collaboration focus
- Goal towards symptom remission, improved functioning, and prevention
- Recognition of the impact of stigma
- Bilingual/bicultural or at least culturally competent in serving minority
  population groups
- Familiarity with community social services (public, private, faith-based)

the mental health care providers, and information was exchanged regarding the patient's medical and psychosocial status. The primary care team focused on preventive care, using US Preventive Services Task Force[54] and VA guidelines.[55]

A total of 120 patients were randomized to receive either this integrated primary care intervention or usual care in the general medical clinics. The average ages of the participants were 45.7 years old (integrated group) and 44.8 years old (usual care). The majority of the patients in both groups had at least one serious psychiatric illness such as post-traumatic stress disorder, substance use disorder, or schizophrenia, or a major affective disorder.

It was found in this study that the integrated model led to improved access to primary care and preventive services, and resulted in significant improvements in health status when compared with a usual care group. Examples include greater likelihood of diabetes screening ($p<0.005$), hepatitis screening ($p<0.003$), cholesterol screening ($p<0.009$), education regarding healthy lifestyle choices ($p<0.01$), and administration of flu vaccine ($p<0.006$). The authors added their impression that some of the factors that led to this improved care included co-location, common chart, enhanced communication, development of shared goals, and sharing of information.

Table 13.3 Acute and maintenance management of depression in the primary care setting

Process of care	Strategies
Recognition and diagnosis	1. Two-question screen Over the past 2 weeks, have you: • Felt little interest or pleasure in doing things? • Felt down, depressed, or hopeless? 2. PHQ-9 initial administration and interpretations 3. Suicide risk assessment
Treatment selection	1. Present treatment options 2. Elicit patient preference
Initial treatment	1. Provide psychoeducation 2. Set self-management goal 3. Explain, recommend, initiate care management
Care management	1. Adherence to treatment initiation 2. Regular monitoring with PHQ-9
Acute phase follow-up	1. Care management with close follow-up and coordinated visits with clinician 2. Modify treatment based on response, or lack thereof
Continuation and maintenance	1. Psychoeducation regarding need for continued treatment after remission 2. Continued treatment with periodic re-evaluations with PHQ-9

PHQ-9, Patient Health Questionnaire.

(Adapted from MacArthur Initiative on Depression and Primary Care.[50])

Conclusion

Several promising collaborative care models have demonstrated that both physical and emotional functioning can improve in patients with co-occurring medical and psychiatric disorders. These studies have further shown that evidence-based depression treatment is feasible in primary care. Whereas the majority of the work has focused on depressive and anxiety disorders, it is likely that similar models can be used to simultaneously address medical and psychiatric comorbidities. For example, Assertive Community Treatment (ACT) teams may be ideally suited to test integration of primary care into a mental health care team that primarily works with patients who have serious mental illness. Given the prevalence of diabetes associated with both the diagnosis of and currently used treatments for schizophrenia, integrating a primary care provider into an ACT team may prove to be particularly beneficial in the management of diabetes in this population of patients. Implementation of these and similar models is likely to have significant impact on improved mental and physical functioning, lower medical utilization and costs, and lower morbidity and mortality.

References

1. Smedley B, Stith A, Nelson A, eds. Unequal Treatment: Confronting Racial and Ethnic Disparities in Healthcare. Washington, DC: National Academies Press, 2003.
2. The WHO World Mental Health Survey Consortium. Prevalence, severity and unmet need for treatment of mental disorders in the World Health Organization world mental health surveys. JAMA 2004; 291: 2581–90.
3. Robins L, Regier D, eds. Psychiatric Disorders in America: The Epidemiologic Catchment Area Study. New York, NY: Free Press, 1991.
4. Kessler RC, McGonagle KA, Zhao S et al. Lifetime and 12-month prevalence of DSM-III-R psychiatric disorders in the United States: results from the National Comorbidity Survey. Arch Gen Psychiatry 1994; 51: 8–19.
5. Druss BG, Bradford WD, Rosenheck RA et al. Quality of medical care and excess mortality in older patients with mental disorders. Arch Gen Psychiatry 2001; 58: 565–72.
6. Osby U, Brandt L, Correia N et al. Excess mortality in bipolar and unipolar disorder in Sweden. Arch Gen Psychiatry 2001; 58: 844–50.
7. Carney RM, Blumenthal JA, Catellier D et al. Depression as a risk factory for mortality after acute myocardial infarction. Am J Cardiol 2003; 92: 1277–81.
8. Frasure-Smith N, Lesperance F, Talajic M. Depression following myocardial infarction: impact on 6-month survival. JAMA 1993; 270: 1819–25.
9. Redelmeier DA, Tan SH, Booth GL. The treatment of unrelated disorders in patients with chronic medical diseases. N Engl J Med 1998; 338: 1516–20.
10. Druss BG, Bradford DW, Rosenheck RA et al. Mental disorders and use of cardiovascular procedures after myocardial infarction. JAMA 2000; 283: 506–11.
11. Graber MA, Bergus G, Dawson JD et al. Effect of a patient's psychiatric history on physicians' estimation of probability of disease. J Gen Intern Med 2000; 15: 204–6.
12. Druss BG, Rosenheck RA, Desai MM et al. Quality of preventive medical care for patients with mental disorders. Med Care 2002; 40: 129–36.
13. Desai MM, Rosenheck RA, Druss BG et al. Mental disorders and quality of diabetes care in the Veterans Health Administration. Am J Psychiatry 2002; 159: 1584–90.
14. Jones LE, Clarke W, Carney CP. Receipt of diabetes services by insured adults with and without claims for mental disorders. Med Care 2004; 42: 1167–75.
15. Frayne SM, Halanych JH, Miller DR et al. Disparities in diabetes care: impact of mental illness. Arch Intern Med 2005; 165: 2631–8.

16. Egede LE, Zheng D, Simpson K. Comorbid depression is associated with increased health care use and expenditures in individuals with diabetes. Diabetes Care 2002; 25: 464–70.
17. Finkelstein EA, Bray JW, Chen H et al. Prevalence and costs of major depression among elderly claimants with diabetes. Diabetes Care 2003; 26: 415–20.
18. Druss BG, Rosenheck RA. Use of medical services by veterans with mental disorders. Psychosomatics 1997; 38: 451–8.
19. Gilbody S, Whitty P, Grimshaw J et al. Educational and organizational interventions to improve the management of depression in primary care: a systematic review. JAMA 2003; 289: 3145–51.
20. Rollman BL, Hanusa BH, Lowe HJ et al. A randomized trial using computerized decision support to improve treatment of major depression in primary care. J Gen Intern Med 2002; 17: 493–503.
21. Bateman DN, Campbell M, Donaldson LJ, Roberts SJ, Smith JM. A prescribing incentive scheme for non-fundholding general practices: an observational study. Br Med J 1996; 313: 535–8.
22. Callahan CM, Hendrie HC, Dittus RS et al. Improving treatment of late life depression in primary care: a randomized clinical trial. J Am Geriatr Soc 1994; 42: 839–46.
23. Brody D, Dietrich AJ, deGruy F 3rd, Kroenke K. The depression in primary care tool kit. Int J Psychiatr Med 2000; 30(2): 99–110.
24. USDHHS. Mental Health: A Report of the Surgeon General. Rockville, MD: US Department of Health and Human Services, Substance Abuse and Mental Health Services Administration, Center for Mental Health Services, National Institutes of Health, National Institute of Mental Health, 1999.
25. Grunebaum M, Luber P, Callahan M et al. Predictors of missed appointments for psychiatric consultations in a primary care clinic. Psychiatr Serv 1996; 47: 848–52.
26. Katon W, Robinson P, Von Korff M et al. A multifaceted intervention to improve treatment of depression in primary care. Arch Gen Psychiatry 1996; 53: 924–32.
27. Katon W, Von Korff M, Lin E et al. Collaborative management to achieve depression treatment guidelines. J Clin Psychiatry 1997; 58(Suppl 1): 20–3.
28. World Health Organization. The Global Burden of Disease. 1996.
29. US Public Health Service, Agency for Health Care Policy and Research. Depression Guideline Panel: Clinical Practice Guideline 2. Treatment of Major Depression, 5: Depression in Primary Care. AHCPR Publication 93-0551. Rockville, MD: US Dept of Health & Human Services, 1993.
30. Spitzer R, Kroenke K, Williams JB. Validation and utility of a self-report version of PRIME-MD: the PHQ Primary Care Study. JAMA 1999; 282: 1737–44.
31. Kominski G, Andersen R, Bastani R et al. UPBEAT: the impact of a psychogeriatric intervention in VA medical centers. Unified Psychogeriatric Biopsychosocial Evaluation and Treatment. Med Care 2001; 39: 500–12.
32. Moye J, Rosansky J, Llorente MD, Jarvik L and the UPBEAT Collaborative Group. Engaging patients in treatment: lessons learned from the UPBEAT Program. Ann Long-Term Care 2001; 9: 61–7.
33. Levkoff S, Chen H, Coakley E et al. Design and sample characteristics of the PRISM-E multisite randomized trial to improve behavioral health care for the elderly. J Aging Health 2004; 16: 3–27.
34. Bartels S, Coakley E, Zubritsky C et al. Improving access to geriatric mental health services: a randomized trial comparing treatment engagement with integrated

versus enhanced referral care for depression, anxiety, and at-risk alcohol use. Am J Psychiatry 2004; 161(8): 1455–62.

35. Dietrich AJ, Oxman TE, Williams JW Jr et al. Re-engineering systems for the treatment of depression in primary care: cluster randomised controlled trial. BMJ 2004; 329: 602.

36. Unützer J, Katon W, Callahan CM et al. Collaborative care management of late-life depression in the primary care setting: a randomized controlled trial. JAMA 2002; 288: 2836–45.

37. Williams JW Jr, Katon W, Lin EH et al. The effectiveness of depression care management on diabetes-related outcomes in older patients. Ann Intern Med 2004; 140: 1015–24.

38. Hunkeler EM, Katon W, Tang L et al. Long-term outcomes from the IMPACT randomized trial for depressed elderly patients in primary care. BMJ 2006; 332: 259–63.

39. Kroenke K, Spitzer RL. The PHQ-9: a new depression diagnostic and severity measure. Psychiatr Ann 2002; 32: 1–7.

40. Unützer J, Choi Y, Cook IA, Oishi S. A web-based data management system to improve care for depression in a multicenter clinical trial. Psychiatr Serv 2002; 53: 671–3.

41. Katon WJ, Von Korff M, Lin EH et al. The Pathways Study: a randomized trial of collaborative care in patients with diabetes and depression. Arch Gen Psychiatry 2004; 61: 1042–9.

42. Lin EH, Katon W, Rutter C et al. Effects of enhanced depression treatment on diabetes self-care. Ann Fam Med 2006; 4(1): 46–53.

43. Bruce ML, Ten Have TR, Reynolds CF et al. Reducing suicidal ideation and depressive symptoms in depressed older primary care patients: a randomized controlled trial. JAMA 2004; 291: 1081–91.

44. Alexopoulos GS, Katz IR, Bruce ML et al. Remission in depressed geriatric primary care patients: a report from the PROSPECT Study. Am J Psychiatry 2005; 162: 718–24.

45. Mulsant BH, Alexopoulos GS, Reynolds CF et al. Pharmacological treatment of depression in older primary care patients: the PROSPECT algorithm. Int J Geriatr Psychiatry 2001; 16: 585–92.

46. Cherry JC, Moffatt TP, Rodriguez C, Dryden K. Diabetes disease management program for an indigent population empowered by telemedicine technology. Diabetes Technol Ther 2002; 4(6): 783–91.

47. Cherry JC, Dryden K, Kobb R et al. Opening a window of opportunity through technology and coordination: a multisite case study. Telemed J E Health 2003; 9(3): 265–71.

48. Huddleston M, Kobb R. Emerging technology for at-risk chronically ill veterans. J Health Qual 2004; 26(6): 12–15, 24.

49. Parks J, Pollack D, eds. Integrating Behavioral Health and Primary Care Services: Opportunities and Challenges for State Mental Health Authorities, 2005. http://www.nasmhpd.org. Last accessed March 29, 2006.

50. The MacArthur Foundation. The MacArthur Foundation Initiative on Depression and Primary Care Tool Kit, 2003. Available at http://www.depression-primarycare.org/clinicians/toolkits. Last accessed March 30, 2006.

51. Druss BG, Rosenheck RA. Locus of mental health treatment in an integrated health care setting. Psychiatr Serv 2000; 51: 890–2.

52. Felker BL, Workman E, Stanley-Tilt C et al. The psychiatric primary care team: a new program to provide medial care to the chronically mentally ill. Med Psychiatry 1998; 1: 36–41.

53. Druss BG, Rohrbaugh RM, Levinson CM, Rosenheck RA. Integrated medical care for patients with serious psychiatric illness: a randomized trial. Arch Gen Psychiatry 2001; 58: 861–8.

54. DiGuiseppi C, Atkins D, Woolf SH, eds. Report of the US Preventive Services Task Force, 2nd edn. Alexandria, VA: International Medical Publishing, 1996.

55. Veterans Health Administration. Health Promotion and Disease Prevention. Washington, DC: Dept of Veterans Affairs, 1996.

Index

Index Page numbers in italic denote tables

abacavir 101
acanthosis nigricans, risk factor
    for DM in general and HIV
    population 91–2
ACE inhibitors 189
advanced glycation endproducts
    (AGEs) 46, 82
aged *see* elderly people
alcohol, limits 120
alcohol abuse, psychosocial
    therapies 205
aldose reductase (AR) inhibitors
    189–90
alphalipoic acid 190
Alzheimer's disease
  association with DM 46–7
  impact of exercise 139–40
  mechanisms linking with DM *45*
amitriptyline *181*, 183
amyotrophy 79
anticonvulsants
  diabetic peripheral neuropathic
      pain *181*, 183–5
  weight gain *124*
antidepressants 35–6, *37*,
    154–60, 198
  depression 35–6, *37*, 154, 198
  eating disorders 202–3

monoamine oxidase inhibitors
    156–7
  impact on DM *162*
  newer *181*
  other 159–60
  serotonin–norepinephrine
      reuptake inhibitors 158–9
  impact on DM *162*
  tricyclics 155–6, *181*, 183
  impact on DM *162*
  side effects *37*, 106–7, 158–9
  treatment of DNP *181*
  weight gain *124*
  see also selective serotonin
      reuptake inhibitors
antidiabetic agents
  injectable 8–9
  oral 7–8, *8*
antipsychotics, atypical (second
    generation) 20–2, 167,
    168–70, 171
  association with DM and DKA
    19, 20–2, 123
  bipolar disorder 165–6
  in HIV-1 infection, risk of
      DM 108–9
  impact on DM *162*
  monitoring 25–6

and nutrition 123
  schizophrenia 167, 168–70
  weight gain risk 123–5, *124*, 160
antipsychotics, typical (first
      generation) 19, 165, 167–8
  schizophrenia 165, 167–8
anxiety disorders
  impact of exercise 138
  and injection avoidance 200
  psychosocial therapies
    CBT and BFRT in adults
        199–201
    children 204
anxiolytics 170–2
  antipsychotics 171
  benzodiazepines 171
  buspirone 172
  hydroxyzine 171
  impact on DM *162*
aripiprazole
  impact on DM *162*
  schizophrenia 168, 169
  weight gain 109
aspirin, and cerebrovascular
    accident risk 105
Assertive Community Treatment
    (ACT) teams 234–5
atazanvir 101
autonomic neuropathy 79
  excise stress test 145

behavioral change, transtheoretical
    model, adherence to exercise 147
behavioral family systems therapy
    (BFST) 209
benzodiazepines
  anxiety disorders 171, 199–200
  impact on DM *162*, 171
  side effects *37*
biofeedback-assisted relaxation
    training (BFRT) 199
biopsychosocial evaluation,
    UPBEAT project 223–5

bipolar disorder 105–6, 161–6
  antipsychotics 165–6
  carbamazepine 164
  lamotrigine 164–5
  lithium 161–3
  mood stabilizers 161–6
  psychotropic drug impact on
      diabetes *162*
  valproic acid/sodium valproate
      163–4
bupropion 159, *181*, 183
  impact on DM *162*
buspirone
  anxiety disorders 172
  impact on DM *162*

capsaicin 188
carbamazepine 164, *181*, 184
  bipolar disorder 164
  impact on DM *162*
  side effects 184
cardiac autonomic neuropathy 79
cardiovascular risk factors,
    and aerobic exercise 132–3, 141
carpal tunnel syndrome 79
cerebrovascular accident,
    complication of DM in HIV-1
      infection 104–5
Charcot's neuroarthropathy 81
chlorpromazine
  abnormal glucose tolerance 19
  schizophrenia 168
  weight gain 23
cholesterol, dietary and LDL,
    management of diabetes *10*, 121
citalopram 157
claudication, and DM 81
clomipramine 155, *181*, 183
clozapine
  glucose intolerance 20–2
  impact on DM *162*
  schizophrenia 168, 169
  weight gain 23, 109, 123

cognitive behavioral therapy
  anxiety disorders 199–201
  for depression 36, 196–7
  eating disorders 201–3
  interpersonal therapy
      196–7, 201
  problem-solving therapy 197–8
cognitive impairment 41–52
  cognition and DM treatment 48–9
  defining 43
  dementia risk and DM 46–7
  epidemiology 41–2
  impact of cognitive decline
      associated with DM 49
  impact of exercise 139–40
  linking mechanisms with type 2
      DM 44–6
    vascular dementia and
        Alzheimer's disease *45*
  types
    MCI and CIND 42–4
    MCI in post-menopausal
        women 48
    risk of decline 47–8
collaborative/integrated care
    219–38
  health care disparities associated
      with psychiatric disorders
      219–21
  Improving Mood-Promoting
      Access to Collaborative
      Treatment (IMPACT study)
      for late-life depression 227–9
  integration of primary care into
      mental health *226*, 232–3
  Pathways Study 229
  Prevention of Suicide in Primary
      Care Elderly: Collaborative
      Trial (PROSPECT) 229–30
  Primary Care Research in
      Substance Abuse and Mental
      Health for the Elderly
      (PRISM-E) 225–6

Re-engineering Systems for the
      Primary Care Treatment
      of Depression (RESPECT-D)
      226–7
  Telemedicine And Care
      Coordination To Improve
      Care for Seniors (TACTICS)
      230–2
  Unified Psychogeriatric
      Biopsychosocial Evaluation
      And Treatment (UPBEAT)
      223–5
coronary artery disease,
    complication of DM in HIV-1
    infection 103–4

dementia
  association with DM 46–7
  impact of exercise 139–40
  see also Alzheimer's disease
depression 29–40, 154–61
  cognitive behavioral therapy
      36, 196–9
    interpersonal therapy 196–7
    problem-solving therapy 197–8
  comorbidities 29
  costs 30
  DM association 30–2
  and glycemic control 206
  in HIV infection, psychiatric
      interventions 106–8
  IMPACT study 227–9
  in children/adolescents 203–4
  management
    acute and maintenance *234*
    antidepressants 35–6,
        37, 154–60, 198
    cognitive behavioral therapy
        36, 196–9
    treatment response rates 198–9
  outcomes and symptoms 32–5
    correlation with glycosylated
        HbA_{1c} *33*

DSM-IV criteria for major
  depression *34*
two-question screen for
  depression *34*
Pathways Study 229
PROSPECT study 229–30
RESPECT-D study 226–7
desipramine 155
diabetes mellitus (DM) 1–16
  anxiety and injection
    avoidance 200
  children/adolescents
    psychosocial factors 205–6
    psychosocial interventions
      207–10
  classification and pathogenesis
    2–3, *10*
  comorbidities 29, 85–6, 106,
    115–16
  definition 1
  diagnosis 3–4
  epidemiology 1–2
  interventional trials 5
  management 5–11
    exercise therapy 133–6
    glycemic goals 5–9, *6, 7*
    injectable therapy 8–9
    LDL cholesterol *10*
    medical nutrition therapy
      117–19
    non-glycemic goals 9–11
    nutrition and physical activity
      6–7, 133–6
    oral antidiabetic agents 7–8, *8*
    psychosocial interventions
      207–10
    recommendations *11*
    self-management 116, 125–6, 133
    treatment goals 4–5
  need for improving care 12–13
  potential linking mechanisms with
    cognitive impairment 44–6

prevention of complications 4–5
prevention trials 11–12
psychosocial factors 205–6
risk of dementia 46–7
risk factors in general population,
  (modifiable) 92–8
  hypertension 93–4
  lipid levels 95
  metabolic syndrome 97–8
  physical activity 96–7
  pregnancy and gestational
    diabetes 92–3
  smoking 96
  weight 92
risk factors in general population,
  (non-modifiable) 90–2
  acanthosis nigricans 91–2
  ethnicity 90
  family history 91
  older age 90
  other clinical conditions
    associated with insulin
    resistance 91–2
  polycystic ovary syndrome 91–2
risk reduction studies 9–11
screening 4
  psychosocial screening 12
types 1 and 2 DM, medical
  nutrition therapy 118–19
diabetic peripheral neuropathic
  pain (DPNP) 75–88, 179–93
  best practices 190
  classification and clinical
    symptoms 76–80, *77–8*
  differential diagnosis *81*
  clinical assessment 82–5
    descriptive, numeric and visual
      pain scales 83
    DPN-specific screening
      instruments 84
    electrodiagnostics 85
    laboratory investigations 84–5

physical examination 84
    risk factors 83
costs 76
education for patient and
    family 86
epidemiology 75–6
in HIV infection 107–8
pathophysiology 81–2
prevention
    foot care 180
    glycemic control 179–80
psychiatric comorbidities 85–6
staging 80–1
symptom management and
    medication trials 180–90
    anticonvulsants 183–5
    antidepressants 183
    disease-modifying treatments
        189–90
    non-opioid medications *181–2*
    non-pharmacologic
        interventions 188–9
    opioids 185–7
    topical agents 188
didanosine 107
doxepin 155
duloxetine 158, *181*, 183
    impact on DM *162*

eating disorders, psychosocial
    therapies 201–3
education of patients 133
efavirenz 101
elderly people
    age as risk factor for DM
        in general and HIV
        population 90
    IMPACT study 227–9
    PRISM-E study 225–6
    PROSPECT study 229–30
    TACTICS project 230–2
    UPBEAT project 223–5

electrodiagnostics, clinical
    assessment of DPNP 85
erythromelalgia 81
escitalopram 157
ethnicity, risk factor for DM
    in general and HIV
        population 90
exercise 131–52
    and cardiovascular risk factors
        132–3, 141
    examples, moderate vs vigorous
        intensity *135*
    impact on DM 6–7, 96–7, 131–6
    impact on psychiatric disorders
        137–40
        anxiety 138
        dementia and cognitive
            impairment 139–40
        schizophrenia 138–9
    recommendations 140–9
        ACSM guidelines for exercise
            testing and prescription *144*
        avoiding hypoglycemia 146
        guidelines *143*
        indications for exercise ECG
            testing *145*
        precautions and
            contraindications 143–6
    resistance training 136, 142
    strategies to improve adherence
        146–9, *148–9*
        self-efficacy/social learning
            model 146–7
        transtheoretical model of
            behavioural change 147
    walking 134–6
    weight loss 134
exercise testing, criteria
    144–5, *145*

family history, risk factor for DM in
    general and HIV population 91

family multisystemic interventions,
children/adolescents with
DM 208–10
family systems therapy (BFST) 209
fatty acids, *trans* 120–1
fluoxetine 157
and HbA$_{1c}$ 35
and weight control 107
foot ulcers
epidemiology 76
prevention 180
see also diabetic peripheral
neuropathic pain (DPNP)
fosamprenavir 101
frequency-modulated electromagnetic
neural stimulation (FREMS) 189

gabapentin, DPN *182*184
gestational diabetes, risk factor
for DM in general and HIV
population 92–3
glitazones (insulin sensitizers) 101
glucose intolerance (impaired
glucose tolerance)
association with (atypical)
antipsychotic medications
19, 20–2
clozapine 20–2
impaired fasting glucose (IFG) *4*
lipodystrophy syndrome, in
HIV-1 infection 95, 98–101
glycemic control
and CBT 199
and depression 206
and exercise 132, 133–6
prevention of diabetic peripheral
neuropathic pain 179–80
and risk of cognitive
impairment 49
glycosylated hemoglobin (HbA$_{1c}$)
correlation with depression *33*, 206
and fluoxetine 35
nutrition therapy 119

haloperidol
impact on DM *162*
schizophrenia 168
Health Buddy appliance and Hero
iCare Desktop 230
health care disparities, associated
with psychiatric disorders
219–21
hepatitis C, HIV-1 co-infection 102
HIV-1 infection 89–114
complications of DM, clinical
management implications
102–5
cerebrovascular accident 104–5
coronary artery disease and
myocardial infarction 103–4
psychiatric implications and
treatments 105–9
atypical antipsychotics, risk of
DM 108–9
comorbidity of DM 106
interventions to reduce
depression and weight
106–8
risk factors in general population
90–8
risk factors specific to HIV-
infected population 98–102
antiretroviral medication
toxicity 101–2
HCV–HIV-1 co-infection 102
lipodystrophy syndrome
98–101
hydroxyzine, anxiety disorders 171
hyperglycemia
as impaired fasting glucose (IFG),
and impaired glucose
tolerance (IGT) *4*
link with depression 196
see also glycemic control
hypertension, risk factor for DM
in general and HIV population
93–4

hypnotics, insomnia 172–3
hypoglycemia, interaction of
        antidepressants with DM
        medications 160

imipramine 155, *181*, 183
impaired glucose tolerance (IGT)
    and impaired fasting glucose
        (IFG) *4*
    prevention/delay of type 2
        DM 11–12
Improving Mood-Promoting
    Access to Collaborative
    Treatment (IMPACT study),
    late-life depression 227–9
information for patients 133
insomnia 172–3
insulin
    action 2–3, *3*
    omission 202
    precautions with physical
        activity 146
insulin resistance
    risk factor for DM in general
        population 91–2
    valproic acid/sodium valproate 163
insulin sensitizers 101
integrated care 219–38
    advantages/disadvantages 222
    integration of primary care into
        mental health 232–3
    mental health in primary care
        221–3, *226*
    see also collaborative care
interferons, increases in general and
    HIV population 95
interpersonal therapy, for
    depression 197

lamotrigine 164–5
    bipolar disorder 164–5
    diabetic peripheral neuropathic
        pain 108, *182*, 184

impact on DM *162*
    and valproic acid/sodium
        valproate 184
LDL cholesterol, management of
    diabetes *10*, 121
lipid levels, risk factor for DM in
    general and HIV population 95
lipodystrophy syndrome, risk
    factor for DM in HIV-1
    infection 95, 98–101
lithium
    bipolar disorder 161–3
    impact on DM *162*
lopinavir–ritonavir 101
loxapine, impact on DM *162*

magnetism, magnetic insoles 189
medical nutrition therapy 117–19
mental health
    integration into primary care
        221–3, *226*
        advantages/disadvantages 222
    primary care, clinician
        competencies *233*
    and primary care providers
        220–1
    PRISM-E study 225–6
metabolic syndrome
    risk factor for DM in general and
        HIV population 97–8
    visceral adiposity vs peripheral
        and central lipoatrophy 100
methadone 186–7
mirtazapine 123–5, 160
    impact on DM *162*
    for insomnia 172
molindone
    impact on DM *162*
    schizophrenia 168
monoamine oxidase inhibitors
    156–7
    side effects *37*
    weight gain 123

mood stabilizers 161–6
  bipolar disorder 161–6
  impact on DM *162*
Morton's neuropathy 81
myocardial infarction, complication
    of DM in HIV-1 infection 103–4

nefadozone 159
  impact on DM *162*
nelfinavir 101
neuropathy *see* diabetic peripheral
    neuropathic pain (DPNP)
nevrapine 101
non-nucleoside reverse transcriptase
    inhibitors (nNRTIs) 89, 101
nortriptyline 155, *181*, 183
  and glucose regulation 35
nucleoside reverse transcriptase
    inhibitors (nRTIs) 89, 101
nutrition 115–29
  dietary composition and
      planning 119–22, *120*
  enhanced adherence factors
      125–6
    food and exercise diary *127*
  interventions 115–17
  medical nutrition therapy 117–19
    benefits 119
    type 1 and 2 DM 118–19
  psychotropic medications, risk of
      weight gain 123–5, *124*

obesity/overweight
  association with schizophrenia
      23, 122
  and insulin resistance 132
  leptin resistance 123–5
  MNT 122
  risk factor for DM in general
      population 92
  waist measurement 23
  see also weight gain

olanzapine
  CATIE trial 22
  hyperglycemia and 21
  impact on DM *162*
  new-onset DM 22
  schizophrenia 169
  weight gain 22–3, 109, 123
    RCT 24
opioids
  diabetic peripheral neuropathic
      pain 185–7
  long-term opioid management *186*
oral glucose tolerance test
    (OGTT) 3
osteoarthritis, in DM 81
oxcarbazepine, DPN *182*, 184
oxidative stress, in DPN 190

pancreas, defects and target tissues
    for insulin action *3*
paroxetine 157
Pathways Study, collaborative
    care 229
percutaneous electrical nerve
    stimulation (PENS) 189
phenothiazines
  impact on DM *162*
  weight gain 123
physical activity *see* exercise
plantar fasciitis 81
polycystic ovary syndrome, risk
    factor for DM in general and
    HIV population 91–2
pregabalin, DPN *182*, 183–4
pregnancy and gestational
    diabetes, risk factor for
    DM in general and HIV
    population 92–3
Prevention of Suicide in
    Primary Care Elderly:
    Collaborative Trial
    (PROSPECT study) 229–30

primary care
  integration of mental health
      care 221–3, *226*
    advantages/disadvantages 222
  Primary Care Research in
      Substance Abuse and
      Mental Health for the Elderly
      (PRISM-E) 225–6
problem-solving therapy, for
    depression 197–8
protease inhibitors (PIs) 89, 101, 102
psychiatric disorders
  associated health care
      disparities 219–21
  comorbidities 29, 115–16
  prevalence, children/adolescents
      with DM 203–6
  psychosocial issues 206–7
psychiatric interventions, reduction
    of depression and weight in
    HIV infection 106–8
psychopharmacologic treatment
    153–77
  *see also specific conditions
      and drugs*
psychosocial factors
  adults with DM 206–7
  children/adolescents 205–6
psychosocial therapies 195–217
  adults with DM 195–203
    depression 195–9
    eating disorders 201–3
    stress and anxiety disorders
        199–201
  children/adolescents with
      DM 203–10
    adherence, control and
        complications 206–7
    anxiety 204
    depression 203–4
    family, peer and multisystemic
        interventions 208–10

stress, coping and
    problem-solving
    interventions 207–8
  substance abuse 205
  see also cognitive behavioral
      therapy
psychotropics
  impact on DM *162*
  risk of weight gain 123–5, *124*, 160
  see also anticonvulsants;
      antidepressants;
      antipsychotics; MAOIs; mood
      stabilizers; SSRIs

quetiapine
  CATIE trial 22
  DM risk 109
  impact on DM *162*
  for insomnia 172
  new-onset DM 22

Re-engineering Systems for the
    Primary Care Treatment of
    Depression (RESPECT-D study)
    226–7
relaxation training,
    biofeedback-assisted
    (BFRT) 199
risperidone
  CATIE trial 22
  DM risk 109
  hyperglycemia and 21
  impact on DM *162*
  new-onset DM 22
  schizophrenia 169
  weight gain 23
ritonavir 101

schizophrenia 17–28, 166–70
  antipsychotics 166–70
  association with DM *19*, 20–2,
      169–70

first-generation 167–8
second-generation 168–70
association with obesity/DM
    18–23, 122, 169–70
and exercise 138–9
as independent risk factor
    for DM 18
prevention, identification and
    management of DM 23–6
selective serotonin reuptake
    inhibitors (SSRIs) 157–8, 161
anxiety disorders 199–200
DNP 183
minimal weight gain *124*, 125
side effects *37*, 107
with tramadol 187
selegiline 156
self-efficacy/social learning model,
    adherence to exercise 146–7
self-management of DM 116,
    125–6, 133
beliefs that increase
    adherence 125–6
serotonin syndrome 107, 187
serotonin–norepinephrine reuptake
    inhibitors 158–9
sertindole, weight gain 23
sertraline 157
sexual dysfunction, men 55–9
depression 57–8
erectile dysfunction, causes 55–7
evaluation 62–3
normal sexual response 53–5
risk factors and physiologic
    component affected *57*
schizophrenia 58–9
treatment 63–4
    apomorphine sublingual
        (Uprima, Ixense,
        Taluvian) 66–7
    intracavernosal injecton
        therapy 67–8

medications associated with *56*
oral medications 65–7
phosphodiesterase type 5
    inhibitors 65–6
prosthesis or penile implants 68
psychotherapy 64
self-administered intraurethral
    therapy 68
vacuum constrictive
    devices 67
sexual dysfunction, women 59–62
causes *54*, 60
    psychological variables *64*
DM 60–2
evaluation 62–3
hypoactive sexual desire
    disorder 69
normal sexual response 53–5
orgasmic disorders 70
sexual arousal disorders 69
sexual pain disorders 70
treatment 63–4, 69–70
    psychotherapy 64
sibutramine 158
smoking, risk factor for DM
    in general and HIV-1
    population 96
social learning model, adherence
    to exercise program 146–7
spinal cord stimulation 188
statins, lipodystrophy syndrome
    100–1
stavudine 101, 107
stimulation-produced
    analgesia 188
stress disorders, psychosocial
    therapies, CBT and BFRT
    in adults 199–201
stress/coping and problem-solving
    interventions, psychosocial
    therapies, children/
    adolescents 207–8

substance abuse
 PRISM-E study 225–6
 psychosocial therapies 205
suicide, PROSPECT study
 229–30

tarsal tunnel syndrome 81
Telemedicine And Care
 Coordination To Improve
 Care for Seniors (TACTICS)
 230–2
 management of depression *234*
 mental health clinician
 competencies *233*
thiothixene, impact on DM *162*
topical agents, diabetic peripheral
 neuropathic pain (DPNP) 188
topiramate, DPN *182*, 185
tramadol 187
trans fatty acids 120–1
transcutaneous electrical nerve
 stimulation (TENS) 188–9
transtheoretical model of
 behavioural change, adherence
 to exercise 147
trazodone 159–60
 impact on DM *162*
 for insomnia 172
trimipramine 155

Unified Psychogeriatric
 Biopsychosocial Evaluation and
 Treatment (UPBEAT project)
 223–5

valproic acid/sodium valproate
 bipolar disorder 163–4
 impact on DM *162*
 insulin resistance 163
 and lamotrigine 184
vascular dementia
 association with DM 46–7
 linking mechanisms with type 2
 DM *45*
venlaxafine 158, *181*, 183
 impact on DM *162*

weight gain
 atypical antipsychotics 171
 control by MNT 122
 exercise strategies 141–3
 in HIV infection, psychiatric
 interventions 106–8
 psychotropic medications
 123–5, *124*
 risk factor for DM in general and
 HIV population 92
 see also obesity/overweight

zalcitabine 107
zidovudine 101
ziprasidone
 CATIE trial 22
 impact on DM *162*
 schizophrenia 168, 169
 weight gain 109
zolpidem
 impact on DM *162*
 for insomnia 172–3